INTERMITTENT FASTING FOR WOMEN

How to Lose Weight, Look Younger and Feel Great (with 65+ Bonus IF Recipes)

Charles Baker

TABLE OF CONTENTS

INTRODUCTION

I am a big believer in putting your health first, but I haven't always felt like this. At the age of 22, I was a college student stuffing my face with every greasy take away food you can think of. I don't think I ever had a home-cooked meal during my first year. Then one day, I got really sick, I thought it was food poisoning, but when I went to the doctors, I was diagnosed with ulcerative colitis which is a form of irritable bowel disease. I was told that there was no cure and that I would be on medication for the rest of my life.

I spent several months going back and forth to the hospital, seeing different doctors and taking various medications (all of which had terrible side effects). I was still eating junk, which is why I wasn't getting any better. After having a bad flare-up that lasted for about a month, I was unable to do anything. My life was on pause, I was using the bathroom up to 30 times a day, I lost a shocking amount of weight, I couldn't eat, and I was terribly depressed, I decided enough was enough. There was no way I was going to live the rest of my life like this.

A friend of mine was into natural health, he was probably one of the healthiest people I knew, he was always speaking to me about my health, but I wasn't interested. I called him for advice; he recommended that I read several books and it was during this time that I stumbled across intermittent fasting, and the rest is history.

I learned everything I could about nutrition and alternative medicine, and completely changed my diet. I cut out all processed foods, sodas and white carbohydrates and focused on eating whole foods. I drank more water and took supplements. Once I started feeling better, I stopped taking my medication, six months into my healthy eating journey, I started intermittent fasting. It made sense to me since my condition was related to digestion that I minimize the amount of times I eat during the day in order to give my digestive system a rest.

I went to the hospital approximately 7 months after starting intermittent fasting, I had a check-up and was told that the medication must be working because there is no more ulcerative colitis in my system. I have never been so happy in my life!

I don't know what has led you to this book, maybe you have had some health challenges, or you just want to lose weight without going on a traditional diet. Whatever the reason, you won't regret your decision to start intermittent fasting, it was the best decision I ever made, and I think it will be for you too!

CHAPTER 1:
INTERMITTENT FASTING AND THE VARIOUS TYPES OF IF

Fasting involves abstinence from food for a certain period of time or significantly reducing your calorie intake. It has been practiced for centuries and there is an avalanche of scientific evidence highlighting it's physical and mental benefits.

Despite the amount of positive information available about fasting, people are still hesitant about participating in the practice. One of the reasons being that society has conditioned us to believe that we are in our healthiest state when we eat three meals a day, and if we don't, we are in some way jeopardising our health and it can lead to things like:

- **Eating Disorders:** Yes, it is true that people who simply decide that they are going to stop eating without a planned strategy are likely to develop eating disorders such as anorexia and bulimia. However, some people have put fasting and eating disorders into the same category and that is not the case. Fasting is a safe and planned way of reaching health goals, whereas an eating disorder is an unhealthy weight loss plan rooted in a compulsive psychological condition.

- **Fluctuations in Sugar and Blood Pressure:** Fasting is still possible for people who suffer from blood related conditions such as diabetes and hypertension. It requires finding the right way to balance the body's natural processes with food consumption. Reduced blood pressure and blood sugar is one of the many benefits of fasting. However, if fasting is not performed with the right amount of preparation and monitoring, it can cause dangerous side effects.

The positive benefits of fasting far outweigh the negative effects, there are several high-tech companies that participate in group fasting with their employees. One of the most popular being the Silicon Valley Group called WeFa.st who participate in monthly meetings and online groups about fasting. They have found that it significantly improves mental clarity. Yoshinoiri Ohsumi, a Japanese biologist received the Nobel Peace Prize in 2016 for his research into autophagy also referred to as cellular self-eating. He found that the body goes through a unique cleansing process during fasting where old cells and cellular debris are disposed of. This process has several health benefits such as slowing down the aging process and eliminating cancer cells.

Even if it is not something we consciously think about, every human being fasts, the simplest definition of the term is the time between the last meal of the day and the first meal of the following day. Therefore, we fast while we are asleep, and rumour has it that the word "breakfast" derives from this. We 'break' our 'fast' when we have our first meal of the morning which is called "breakfast." Fasting is abstaining from eating for a period of time to allow the body to renew itself.

Intermittent Fasting - What is it?

Intermittent fasting (IF), is a planned form of cyclical fasting, it involves eating between certain times and sticking to it. Some people consume a specific diet during their eating window, I will discuss this in a later chapter. Intermittent fasting is NOT a diet, it changes when you eat and not what you eat. There are some major benefits associated with changing when you eat, it's the most effective way of getting lean without going on an extreme diet or reducing your calories down to nothing (depending on the fast you choose). Additionally, IF is a great way to get lean while keeping muscle mass.

One of the main reasons why people use intermittent fasting is to lose fat (I'll go into that later). Most importantly, intermittent fasting is one of the easiest ways to maintain good weight and shed bad weight because it requires very little change to your regular eating schedule or food consumption. This is extremely beneficial because it means that it's simple enough for you to actually do it, but also very effective at the same time.

<u>There are several types of intermittent fasts, these include</u>:

The 5:2 Twice a Week Method: This type of intermittent fast involves eating 500 calories a day twice a week, you consume a normal diet during the other five days of the week. During fasting days, the diet includes one 200 calorie meal and one 300 calorie meal. It is also important to focus on high-protein and high-fiber foods to keep calories low and to keep you full during the fast. There are no restrictions on the two days chosen as long as you have a day's break in between fasting. For example, you can fast on Monday and Wednesday, or Tuesday and Thursday. On non-fasting days, you should also make sure that you eat the same amount of foods you normally would.

Time Restricted Eating: Placing a time restriction on eating involves eating between certain times. For example, you can choose not to eat for 16 hours of the day and eat any time between an eight-hour window. This method is popular because as I have mentioned, most people fast during their sleep anyway, and so it only involves skipping breakfast and then eating at lunch time. The most common ways for time restricted eating include:

- **16/8 Method:** Eating between 11 a.m. and 7 p.m. or noon and 8 p.m.
- **14/10 Method:** Eating between 10 a.m. and 8 p.m.

You can repeat this method of intermittent fasting as many times as you wish throughout the week. Some people have made it a lifestyle choice, the right fasting window for you will depend on your schedule and how your body works. For those wanting to try out intermittent fasting for the first time, this is the safer option.

Alternate Day Fasting: This type of fast involves changing your fast every other day. For example, you might consume 500 calories on your fasting day or a percentage of your normal calorie intake. On non-fasting days, you revert back to your normal diet. The alternate day fasting also has strict variations that involve not consuming any calories on your fasting days.

The Eat Stop Eat Method: Also known as the 24 hours fast, this method involves not eating anything for a full 24 hours. It is performed once or twice per week and typically involves fasting from dinner time to dinner time, from lunch time to lunch time or from breakfast time to breakfast time. However, people often report side effects such as low energy, hunger, irritability, headaches and fatigue while on this type of fast.

INTERMITTENT FASTING IS NOT A QUICK FIX

No matter what type of diet you are on, it all comes down to how much and the quality of calories you are consuming. The long-term effects of intermittent fasting are still under investigation; however, it is important that you eat a well-balanced and healthy diet while intermittent fasting. You will often hear so called gurus stating that they eat what they like during their eating window and that includes junk foods and high fat foods. Well, that defeats the purpose of intermittent fasting because overall, the main aim is to improve your health and experience the benefits associated with this way of eating.

CHAPTER 2:
WHY INTERMITTENT FASTING IS SUPERIOR

With so many people speaking out about the health benefits of intermittent fasting, the medical field have been forced to pay attention, and a growing body of research has discovered that timing is one of the most important factors in eating, and that intermittent fasting can be a sustainable, realistic and effective approach for weight loss as well as other health benefits.

It's a Simple Solution to Dieting: Most people fail miserably when they attempt to go on a diet because they are often extremely restrictive and require a dramatic change in your eating habits. Intermittent fasting isn't a diet, and therefore, it doesn't require a change in behaviour which is where the majority of people struggle. For example, one study found that obese adults found intermittent fasting extremely effective because participants were able to adapt to their new eating schedules in a relatively short period of time.

Dr. Michael Eades tried intermittent fasting for himself and highlighted that diets are easy in theory but difficult in practice. When we find a diet appealing, the majority of us think about trying it out because the thought of it seems easy. He mentions that his eating habit is a low carbohydrate diet, but if he were to go on a low-fat diet, he would find it difficult because he would want to eat the foods that he normally consumes such as meat and eggs. On the other hand, intermittent fasting seems difficult when you think about it, but once you start there are so many benefits, you don't want to stop. Outside of the health benefits, it frees you from having to think about what to eat three times a day, it gives you additional time to do other things, and you save money on food expenses.

As stated, I am an advocate of intermittent fasting, I practice it myself and I would say that the simplicity of this way of eating and the fact that it doesn't require a massive behaviour change is one of the best reasons to consider IF.

Reduces Your Risk of Cancer: There has been a limited amount of research on this, so I am not claiming that it is a fact. However, there have been several studies done on the relationship between fasting and cancer and there are many positive conclusions. One study of 10 cancer patients found that the effects of chemotherapy were reduced by fasting prior to treatment. Another study also supports this finding after it found that alternate day fasting before chemotherapy resulted in fewer deaths and better cure rates.

Finally, an evaluation of several studies on disease and fasting discovered that not only does fasting reduce the risk of cancer, it also reduces the risk of cardiovascular disease.

Increases Life Span: It is no secret in the science community that restricting calories increases lifespan. This makes sense from a logical standpoint because when the body goes into starvation mode, it finds a way to live longer. The problem is that no one wants to starve themselves to live longer; the good news is that with intermittent fasting, you don't have to starve yourself to experience the same benefits.

In 1945, it was discovered that intermittent fasting increased the life span of mice. A recent study also found that IF has a positive effect on lifespan.

Intermittent Fasting Simplifies Your Life: As discovered by Dr. Eades intermittent fasting makes your days a lot simpler. I am a fan of reducing stress, simplicity and behaviour change and intermittent fasting provides me with an additional element of simplicity giving me one less thing that I need to worry about. Think about it, some people (especially mothers) spend the majority of their days in the kitchen preparing breakfast, lunch and dinner. Unless you have enough money to hire a chef, you are going to spend way too much time cooking. And if you are ambitious like me, and you value time, finding the time to prepare meals can become stressful.

With intermittent fasting, I don't think about breakfast, I have a cup of green tea and get on with my day. I don't mind cooking and I like eating, but I did find that making three meals a day was a drain on my time and I would meal prep on Sundays to cut down on cooking throughout the week. Since I no longer eat breakfast, it's one less meal I've got to think about.

Side Effects of Intermittent Fasting

If I were to leave this section out, I would be doing my readers a huge disservice. Although I am an advocate of intermittent fasting and research suggests that there are many benefits associated with the practice, there have also been many reported cases of negative side effects. I am including what I have found in my studies so that you can make an informed and intelligent decision as to whether you want to go ahead with intermittent fasting or not.

Mood Changes: Intermittent fasting is a restrictive diet, and when you first start, it is possible that you will experience a change in mood. On the other hand, some people do report a boost of motivation and energy once their body adjusts to the diet. However, if you begin to feel anxious, depressed or discouraged because of IF, it's important to stop and get in contact with a nutrition coach or a registered dietician to help you develop a fasting schedule that better suits your body and mind.

Sleep Disturbances: Some people have reported improved sleep patterns during intermittent fasting. This might be due to the way IF helps to control late night snacking habits which makes it difficult to fall asleep because the body is still trying to digest the cookies you ate at 10 p.m.

However, some research suggests the opposite, an article in the journal Nature and Science of Sleep states that daytime fasting causes a reduction in rapid eye movement (REM) sleep. There are several benefits linked to getting enough REM sleep including better concentration, cognitive processing and memory. If you find it difficult to sleep after you start intermittent fasting, take a break and speak to a professional to ensure that you are not damaging your health.

Unhealthy Diet: The main concern is that it can trigger binge eating behaviour because of how hungry you feel after the fast. It can lead to you eating way more than your recommended daily calorie requirement. If you start intermittent fasting and experience this problem, go and see a dietician to determine the most effective way of eating to fuel your body with the right nutrients throughout the day instead of during a specific window.

Constipation: Intermittent fasting is not the cause of constipation; however, any diet will give you an upset stomach if you are not getting enough fiber, protein, vitamins and fluid. Regardless of what you are eating, it is important to stay hydrated throughout the day. Most people drink with their meals, and it's easy to abandon your fluid intake when taking a break from eating for 16 hours. If you start finding it difficult to go to the toilet during intermittent fasting, there could be more going on than you not drinking enough water. A professional will help you decide what nutrients you need to consume more of to get you regular again.

Changes in Menstrual Cycle: One of the results of intermittent fasting is sudden weight loss. Women who lose large amounts of weight in a short period of time or who do not consume enough calories throughout the day may find that they experience a slowdown with their menstrual cycle or that it stops completely. According to the Mayo Clinic, women who are extremely underweight are susceptible to amenorrhoea which is a loss of menstruation. Being underweight, or sudden weight loss can interrupt your normal hormone cycle which leads to missed periods. So, although you may be excited about the way intermittent fasting has helped you lose weight, you may also be putting your body at risk by failing to provide it with its required calorie intake.

Hair Loss: Depriving the body of nutrients, or the sudden weight loss, especially B vitamins and proteins can cause hair loss. It is important to mention that although intermittent fasting doesn't lead to the body losing nutrients, it is more difficult to consume a balanced diet when you are eating for the entire day within a few short hours. If you start noticing bald patches, or that more hair than normal is falling out when you brush it, speak to your doctor to get advice on how to get more nutrients into your diet.

Low Blood Sugar: If you experience dizziness, headaches or nausea during intermittent fasting, that is a sign that it is having a negative effect on your blood sugar. Experts suggest that for this reason, diabetics should avoid any type of fasting as it can lead to hypoglycaemia which is a dangerous condition for anyone suffering from thyroid or insulin problems.

Food Obsessions: All restrictive diets have the potential to affect your relationship with food. While some people enjoy the strict nature of intermittent fasting, others may find that they spend too much time focusing on how many calories they are getting and what they can eat. According to The National Eating Disorders Associations, an obsession with the quality and quantity of your daily food intake can lead to a condition called orthorexia which means that you focus so much on healthy eating that it begins to have a negative effect on your overall well-being. This is not the point of dieting; it is to assist you in building a positive relationship with food and not a negative one.

Brain Fog or Fatigue: If you find that you are making careless mistakes or becoming extremely tired throughout the day because of brain fog and fatigue, it's a sign that you are not eating the right foods during your fasting hours or that intermittent fasting is not ideal for your lifestyle. Pay close attention to what you eat during your non-fasting hours to ensure you are fuelling your body with the foods that will make you feel strong and healthy.

Feeling Hangry (no it's not a typo): The word "hangry" has yet to find its way into the English dictionary, but it is a popular term in the IF community. It is the feeling of irritability, grouchiness or grumpiness because you are not able to eat when the body is telling you it's hungry. It takes a lot of practice to train your body to abstain from food for several hours, especially when you have been so used to eating at certain times. You should bear in mind that there are some people who will never get used to eating during certain hours alone. In theory, if you are getting the right amounts of protein later in the day, you shouldn't be hungry when you wake up in the morning. But if you are, it is an indication that you need to make some adjustments to your diet during your eating hours. For some people, especially those who go to the gym a lot, intermittent fasting might not be a good idea. But there is nothing stopping you from testing it out to see how your body responds.

CHAPTER 3:
INTERMITTENT FASTING - A POWERFUL WEIGHT LOSS TOOL

Okay, so you have read about some of the impressive health benefits associated with intermittent fasting; the question is, what is the science behind these theories and what happens to the genes and hormones when we fast?

Intermittent Fasting Burns Fat and Not Sugar: During fasting, instead of burning sugar for energy, it burns fat, and this is what improves brain function and accelerates weight loss. Like a car, the body can't function without fuel, it gets its fuel from fasting. The stomach breaks down carbohydrates into sugar during digestion and your cells use it for energy. You will also hear this energy referred to as glucose. When the cells don't use all the available glucose, the remainder is stored as fat.

When the body is in fasting mode, the cells use fat as the primary fuel source instead of glucose. As a result, your fat stores - mainly triglycerides, are burnt up for energy which is why many studies have found that intermittent fasting leads to weight loss as well as reducing the risk of cardiovascular disease. Some experts suggest that this shift takes place as early as 10 to 16 hours after starting a fast. The body doesn't start breaking down protein to use as fuel until around the third day of fasting. This means that intermittent fasting can help the body maintain muscle mass at the same time as reduce fat.

When fat stores are used for energy, ketones are released into the bloodstream. Ketones are fatty acids that play an important role in weight loss, but research also suggests that they preserve brain function. Therefore, intermittent fasting may offer some security against Alzheimer's disease, epileptic seizures and other neurodegenerative conditions. For example, one study found that older adults suffering from a slight cognitive impairment experienced improved memory within six weeks due to a boost in ketones. These benefits might be the result of ketones triggering the release of brain-derived neurotrophic factor (BDNF), which enhances neural connections, especially in the areas associated with learning and memory. Studies also suggest that intermittent fasting encourages the growth of new nerve cells in the brain.

Improves Insulin Sensitivity and Lowers Insulin: Fasting causes a drop in insulin levels and an increase in norepinephrine and the human growth hormone. This protects the body against chronic disease and accelerates the weight loss process. In other words, when we eat, the body is flooded with insulin, and there is a massive decrease when we fast. Insulin determines whether excess glucose is stored in the body as fat - this is another reason why intermittent fasting has such a powerful effect on weight loss. Research suggests that IF improves insulin sensitivity as well as reduce hyperinsulinemia which is a condition where there is more insulin in the blood than glucose. Several studies have found that intermittent fasting has reduced and reversed diabetes in rats.

Research has also found that low insulin levels cause a rise in FoxO transcription factors which control the genes responsible for metabolism. Ultimately, this process may transform gene expression in favour of longevity and healthy aging. Research also suggests that intermittent fasting lowers insulin-like growth factor 1, a genetic marker for diseases such as cancer.

Increase in Human Growth Hormone: Studies reveal that fasting stimulates the release of the human growth hormone (HGH). This is significant because the body produces less HGH as we age which is associated with a loss of muscle mass and in increase in fat tissue which explains why most people start putting on weight as they age. Therefore, the increase in HGH is also associated with maintaining muscle mass at the same time as losing weight.

Improves Circadian Rhythm: Some studies suggest that intermittent fasting helps improve sleep patterns. The circadian cycle in humans relates to the light and dark cycle; evolution has programmed the body to eat during the daytime (light cycle) and fast during the night-time (dark cycle). When we conform to this natural cycle, the metabolism is more efficient. However, our modern lifestyles have disrupted this cycle because we now spend more time awake and active during the dark cycle. A lot of people are eating when they should be sleeping and fasting; this disruption has caused reduced metabolic efficiency and overeating.

Following a time restricted approach to intermittent fasting may improve metabolism and regulate circadian rhythms. Research suggests that synchronizing our biological clock with our eating patterns can lead to reduced obesity and improved weight regulation. Studies also suggest that through this harmonization, intermittent fasting also restores beneficial gut bacteria and encourages the normal expression of the genes responsible for liver health.

Boosts the Cells Resiliency and Health: During intermittent fasting, your cells get a bit stressed out (in a good way), as a result, they build resilience which makes them stronger. Mark Mattison from the National Institute of Aging states that the stress the cells are placed under during intermittent fasting is similar to the stress placed on the heart and muscles during exercise. It shocks the system and causes the body to become stronger over time.

Boosts Norepinephrine: This neurotransmitter helps the body break down fuel and fat and therefore has a positive impact on the body's metabolism.

CHAPTER 4:
MYTHS AND MISCONCEPTIONS – DEBUNKING INTERMITTENT FASTING

Despite the fact that intermittent fasting has become extremely popular over the years, there are still many myths and misconceptions floating around, many of which have been circulated by people with no credentials and have no real understanding of the practice. Nevertheless, some of these myths have caused those who hear them to abandon the idea of intermittent fasting altogether. In this chapter, I am going to challenge some of those myths and provide scientific evidence to bolster my claims.

Intermittent Fasting Causes Overeating

In some circles it is believed that intermittent fasting causes you to overeat during the eating window. Although you might eat more calories than you would during one meal after the fast, there is no evidence to suggest that it leads to overcompensation.

One study found that participants who fasted for 24 hours consumed approximately 500 extra calories the following day, which was a lot less than the 2,400 calories they did not eat during the fast. Since fasting causes a reduction in insulin levels at the same time as boosting human growth hormone levels, norepinephrine levels and metabolism, intermittent fasting does not make you gain fat but lose it.

It was determined in a review that a fast of 2-24 weeks caused average belly fat and weight loss of 3-8% and 4-7% respectively. Therefore, it could be that intermittent fasting is one of the most effective weight loss tools.

Intermittent Fasting Makes You Lose Muscle
The myth is that fasting causes the body to burn muscle for fuel. Although this is what happens when you go on a typical diet, there is no evidence to suggest that this process also takes place with intermittent fasting. In fact, evidence suggests that the practice is highly effective for building muscle.

One study discovered that continuous calorie restriction and intermittent fasting led to the same amount of weight loss, but there was less reduction in muscle mass with intermittent fasting. Another study found that participants who consumed all their calories during one meal experienced a modest increase in muscle mass.

Additionally, intermittent fasting is extremely popular amongst body builders, they find that it helps maintain a low body fat percentage as well as maintain muscle mass.

The Body is Only Capable of Using a Limited Amount of Protein Per Meal

Rumour has it that the body is only capable of digesting 30 grams of protein per meal, and that in order to maximize muscle gain you should eat every 2-3 hours. However, science does not support this claim. Studies suggest that there is no connection between muscle mass and eating frequent doses of protein. When it comes to protein, what's important is the amount consumed and not how often.

Intermittent Fasting Causes the Body to go Into Starvation Mode

One popular argument against intermittent fasting is that it causes the body to go into starvation mode. This then shuts down the metabolism and prevents the body from burning fat. Although it is true that long term weight loss can limit the number of calories the body burns overtime, this is not caused by intermittent fasting, it happens regardless of the weight loss method used.

There is no evidence to support the claim that intermittent fasting leads to a greater loss in calories than any other weight loss strategies. However, evidence does suggest that short-term fasting can cause an increase in metabolic rate as a result of the significant increase of blood levels of norepinephrine. It is the hormone responsible for stimulating the metabolism and instructing the fat cells to break down body fat.

Studies suggest that participants who fasted for up to 48 hours experienced a boost in their metabolism by 3.6-14%. However, it is also important to mention that fasting for longer periods than this can reverse the effects and cause a decrease in metabolism.

One study discovered that fasting every other day for 22 days caused an average of 4% loss of fat mass but there was no reduction in metabolic rate.

It is Good for Your Health to Eat Often
It is believed that eating on a regular basis is good for your health and the less you eat, the more damage you are causing to the body. However, studies fail to support this claim and suggests that short-term fasting induces autophagy which is a cellular repair process, it protects against cancer, Alzheimer's and

aging. On the other hand, some studies suggest that eating often and snacking can increase your risk of disease and cause a number of health issues.

For example, in one study it was discovered that consuming several high calorie meals led to an increase in liver fat which increased the risk of fatty liver disease. Additionally, other studies indicate that people who eat often have an increased risk of colorectal cancer.

The Brain Needs a Continuous Supply of Dietary Glucose

One argument suggests that a failure to eat carbohydrates every few hours will cause the brain to stop operating. This idea originates from the belief that the only fuel the brain can use is glucose. However, the body is capable of producing the glucose it requires through a process called gluconeogenesis. Even on very low-carb diets, starvation or long-term fasting, the body produces ketones from dietary fats. As you have read, ketone bodies have the ability to feed parts of the brain which significantly reduces its glucose requirement.

Some people do report feeling shaky after extended periods without food, if you experience this, you should carry a selection of healthy snacks that you can eat when you need to.

Frequent Meals Encourage Weight Loss

Since eating often doesn't boost your metabolism, neither does it encourage weight loss, this claim goes unsubstantiated. A study of 16 obese adults compared the effects of eating 3 and 6 meals per day. The study found no difference in appetite, fat loss or weight.

Some people have stated that eating frequent meals helps them stick to a healthy diet, if you feel that it helps you eat less junk food and fewer calories, experts advise that you stick to eating frequent meals.

Eating Often Reduces Hunger

Many people believe that frequent eating helps reduce excessive hunger and cravings. However, some studies support this claim, but others don't. One study found that eating between 3 and 6 meals high in protein per day effectively reduced hunger. But it is also important to mention that how the body responds will depend on the individual. If you find that eating often reduces cravings then that is what you should do, but the research does not support that this is the case for everyone who eats often.

Eating Often Boosts Metabolism

It has been argued that eating often increases your metabolic rate and causes the body to burn more calories. While it is true that the body burns calories when it is digesting food, it does not mean that it will increase your metabolism. The reason being is that what's important is not the number of meals you eat, but how many calories you consume.

If you eat six five calorie meals, it is no different than eating three 1,000 calorie meals. Several studies prove that increasing or decreasing the number of meals eaten has no effect on the calories burnt.

Not Eating Breakfast Makes You Put on Weight

The myth that breakfast is the most important meal of the day has been around for several years. The main belief is that skipping breakfast causes excessive cravings and hunger which leads to weight gain. A 16-week study with 283 overweight and obese participants found that there was no difference between those who ate breakfast and those who missed it.

Therefore, in general, breakfast has no effect on your weight although results may vary depending on the individual. On the other hand, several studies indicate that those who lose weight over the long term typically eat breakfast.

It is also important to mention that research suggests that children who eat breakfast in the morning tend to have a better academic performance in school. Therefore, before you decide to skip breakfast, you should take your individual needs into consideration.

There are so many myths about intermittent fasting that it would be impossible for me to document them all here, but those I have listed are the most popular. What I would advise is that when conducting research, you do so using authoritative sources that provide evidence from academic sources to ensure that the information you are reading is accurate.

CHAPTER 5: INTERMITTENT FASTING FOR WOMEN

In general, women who choose to fast should pay attention to any symptoms that make them feel uncomfortable. Your body will alert you if something is wrong, and if you really don't feel right, stop fasting and book an appointment with your doctor.

Both men and women have a good response to fasting; however, the evidence suggests that women typically experience a better response to fasting because they spend more time dieting. During the first two weeks, women will lose less weight than men, but within four to six weeks, they catch up. Some women don't lose any weight when intermittent fasting; rather, they experience increased muscle mass and their clothes start to fit better. It is important to remember that the number on a weighing scale does not indicate successful weight loss.

Women who fast report positive hormonal changes, they experience better sex lives, elevated moods, less brain fog, and a reduction in negative premenstrual symptoms. As you have read, the process of autophagy protects the body against cancer by eliminating mutated and damaged cells which reduces the risk of cervical, ovarian and breast cancer in women.

Women, Obesity and Intermittent Fasting

Whether male or female, there is nothing good about obesity; but it is especially dangerous for women because of the effect that it has on female hormones. Fat cells produce estrogen, and when there is too much estrogen in the body it prevents the efficient production of progesterone and upsets the hypothalamic-pituitary-gondal axis (HPG axis). Although these glands each have their own individual functions, they often act in concert; therefore, endocrinologists and physiologists find it convenient to refer to them as one single system. The HPG axis is responsible for regulating female reproductive ability and hormones, when it is disrupted, it can cause estrogen dominance. This is a hormonal imbalance that leads to issues such as difficulty sleeping, weight gain, problems with ovulation, cysts, endometriosis, miscarriages, heavy periods, absent or irregular periods and poor mood control.

Another negative consequence associated with obesity is that it causes insulin resistance; this leads to an increase in insulin production and insulin resistance. Too much insulin stimulates the release of the hunger hormones leptin and ghrelin which leads to the desire to eat more with the end result being excessive weight gain. It is a vicious cycle that many women struggle with. Intermittent fasting can resolve these issues by increasing insulin sensitivity which will regulate hunger. Additionally, IF will burn the fat responsible for producing too much estrogen.

Women and Cholesterol

According to research, women need cholesterol more than men. Cholesterol is the wax that coats the veins and the body uses it to produce vitamin D, bile acids, progesterone and estrogen. While we all need vitamin D and bile acids; estrogen and progesterone are essential to female reproductive health. Without them, women will not be able to ovulate, release eggs or get pregnant. Since women need cholesterol, their bodies tend to produce excess. After menopause the majority of women suffer from high cholesterol which can clog the arteries and eventually cause serious heart trouble. High cholesterol can also cause visceral fat which coats the organs and prevents them from functioning effectively.

Fasting and its Effect on Hormones

Women are more sensitive to fasting than men because they have more of the hormone kisspeptin. It is also believed that women have more cortisol which has a negative effect on their sleep cycle. Both of these hormones can disrupt the HPG axis which as you have read has an adverse effect on the production of progesterone and estrogen.

Therefore, women should ease their way into fasting and only engage in moderate exercise whilst they are fasting and on their period. In this way, the negative side effects of intermittent fasting are reduced. Typically, when women get used to fasting, they find that their hormones are balanced which leads to better sleep patterns and it improves their ability to handle stress because the HPG axis has been balanced.

The Best Approach to Fasting for Women

The most effective fasting method for women is the 5:2 approach. That is to fast for 24 hours twice a week, when they are not fasting, they should consume high amounts of healthy protein sources from nuts, plants and animals. Women should also ease into fasting by starting with a 12 hour fast, then moving onto the 16:8 method, and then the 5:2 approach. Be sure to have bone broth available for additional protein and to reduce cravings. Don't exercise if you are not feeling strong enough or perform a light workout routine. During your period, consume additional iron and a minimum of 500 calories; sufficient calories is essential to preventing hormonal disruption.

Symptoms to Pay Attention to
There are several possible side effects associated with intermittent fasting. However, women are susceptible to some additional side effects and if you experience any of them, stop fasting immediately and book an appointment with your doctor.

- Severe stomach pain
- Vomiting
- Fainting
- Dizziness
- Migraines
- Heavy periods
- Unusually painful periods
- The absence of a period if you are not pregnant
- Skin rashes
- Extreme weight loss
- Weight gain
- Hair loss

- Pale skin
- Bleeding during sex
- Unusual pelvic pain

Fasting During Menstruation

Some women experience a disruption to their menstrual cycle while fasting, this can mean that your period will stop completely for a short time. However, once the body starts getting the nutrition it needs and gets used to fasting, your periods will return. Fasting puts pressure on the body, and this is how it reacts to the stress that has been caused. It is a natural by-product of fasting and experts advise that it is nothing to worry about. If a healthy diet is practiced during the fasting window, IF will eventually lead to improved hormonal balance in women. When your periods stop, it is a sign that you are in the adjustment phase.

Some women who practice intermittent fasting may experience hormonal issues that lead to hair loss, pale skin and the early onset of menopause. These problems typically do not last for more than a few months if intermittent fasting is followed properly. Therefore, it is important to consume a well-balanced diet with sufficient calories during your eating window. You should also take a good multivitamin and pay careful attention to your body because if anything is wrong it will let you know.

As mentioned, not all women experience a loss of menstruation during fasting. Many women have reported less cramps and lighter periods when they are fasting. It is normal for women to feel hungrier during their period, so you might want to switch up your fasting days during your time of the month.

CHAPTER 6:
INTERMITTENT FASTING FOR WOMEN OVER 50

Women begin experiencing menopause between the ages of 45 and 55. However, whether they are going through menopause or not, there are certain hormonal changes that start taking place at the age of 50. After women reach menopause their risk of heart attack increases because the body stops producing as much estrogen. Estrogen helps to keep the arteries supple, and lower levels may explain why bad cholesterol and high blood pressure tend to rise during this time. Furthermore, late peri and post menopause are associated with more deposits of fat around the heart which a 2015 study reports increased the risk of heart disease by 54 percent.

One way to mitigate this is to get rid of fat around the abdomen. The fat in this region is especially toxic because it produces compounds such as cytokines, they are inflammatory proteins which have been linked to heart disease, type 2 diabetes and insulin resistance.

One solution is to start hormone replacement therapy; however, timing is imperative because if you start hormone replacement therapy while going through perimenopause, it can help prevent you from developing fat around the midriff. However, it may be too late if you wait until you've passed menopause. Deborah Clegg, PhD, a professor of biomedical sciences at Cedars-Sinai in Los Angeles advises that if women don't want hormone replacement therapy, they should commit to consuming a diet low in saturated fat and sugar and rich in lean protein, fish, nuts, whole grains, vegetables and fruits as well as commit to regular exercise.

Urinary Incontinence: Basically, women start wetting themselves when menopause peaks because estrogen levels decline. When there are low levels of estrogen in the body it causes the muscles in the vaginal and urinary tract to weaken making women susceptible to leakage. Additionally, weight gain increases the chances of urinary incontinence because of the increased pressure on the bladder and surrounding muscles.

An effective solution for this problem is vaginal estrogen, it is available in the form of a suppository, cream or a vaginal ring placed around the genital area to boost estrogen levels in those tissues. Not only will it reduce incontinence, but it will also ease symptoms such as irritation, itching and vaginal dryness. The additional estrogen helps balance levels of vaginal bacteria which keeps the vaginal pH at a normal level and reduces the risk of getting both urinary tract and yeast infections.

If vaginal estrogen doesn't appeal to you, pelvic floor exercises can also help to tighten the muscles in the bladder area. A clinical trial conducted in Canada discovered that 75 percent of participants experienced a reduction in urinary incontinence after 12 weeks of physical therapy sessions that involved pelvic floor exercises.

Vitamin D: You will have heard vitamin D referred to as 'the sunshine vitamin' because the body produces it when the skin is exposed to the sun. Vitamin D acts as a hormone to help maintain your muscle, nerve function and immune system. It also regulates the immune system and strengthens the bones. Studies suggest that vitamin D plays a role in protecting the brain against disorders such as dementia.

The risk of vitamin D deficiency increases with age because the skin becomes less capable of using sun rays to make vitamin D. Therefore, consider taking a vitamin D supplement since you may not be able to get enough from UV rays and food alone. The Albert Einstein College of Medicine recommends that women in their 50's and 60's should take around 600 IUs per day. One study revealed that participants who took 2000 IUs per day for two weeks experienced reduced levels of the stress hormone cortisol, lower blood pressure and better fitness performance than the placebo group. However, experts do not recommend taking more than 2000 IUs because some studies have found a link between high dosages of vitamin D and developing kidney stones.

Bone Loss: Bone loss is another problem that women experience when they reach menopause. However, it is possible to slow the rate of bone loss by incorporating weight bearing exercises into a workout routine. Weight bearing assists in maintaining bone density, but there will still be a decline in bone mass due to hormonal changes. This is why women over the age of 50 need to increase their intake of vitamin D, calcium and protein. Experts advise that menopausal women consume 1,200 mg of calcium per day, you can get 300 mg from one cup of non-fat milk and additional dairy sources include low-fat cottage cheese and yogurt. Non-dairy sources include breakfast cereal, soymilk and fortified orange juice.

Friendly Fats: Unsaturated and nutrient rich fats are essential to healthy aging. They protect against stroke, heart attack and coronary artery disease. They also protect the myelin coating of nerve fibers which enables them to work effectively. Fat also keeps the body from drying out and the skin supple. You can compare it to putting lotion on the body from the inside out.

Women over the age of 50 can increase their omega 3 fatty acid intake by eating three servings of sardines, mackerel, salmon or tuna per week. Omega 3 is also available in avocados, oils such as sesame, walnut and olive oil and nuts and seeds such as flaxseed, chia, pumpkin, sesame and sunflower.

Additional Protein: Women over the age of 50 should consume approximately 5 to 6 ounces of protein per day. Preferred meat sources include pork loin with the outer layer of fat removed, skinless chicken breast, venison, bison and lean beef. For vegetarians and vegans, protein is available in lentils, kidney beans, pinto beans and soybeans. They are also high in fiber which helps keep bad cholesterol levels low.

Signs of Nutrient Deficiencies: Women in their 50's who are not eating a balanced diet or getting the right amount of nutrients from foods will experience nutrient deficiencies. They may experience bleeding gums, frequent injuries, fractures, forgetfulness and fatigue.

Consuming a nutrient rich diet as well as engaging in regular physical activity can help combat tiredness; vitamin D and calcium can enhance bone density; iron and vitamin C can prevent bleeding gums and vitamin B12 can improve memory. If you are experiencing any of the above symptoms, it is essential that you go to the doctors and have your vitamin D and B12 levels checked.

Another symptom of nutrient deficiency that is easily prevented is drinking enough water to combat dehydration. Older people lose sensitivity in their thirst mechanisms, and as a result, they do not realize they are dehydrated. The Mayo Clinic recommends drinking 2.2 liters or 9 cups of water per day.

Fasting During Menopause
There are a limited number of studies about the effects of fasting on menopausal women. Dr. Becky Gillapsy conducted an evaluation on fasting, aging,

and women's health and she discovered that menopausal women did not have a different experience than non-menopausal women during fasting.

Menopause causes the body to stop producing certain hormones, it accelerates aging and other health problems. However, fasting assists the body in mitigating these issues through autophagy. Menopausal women are at a higher risk of breast cancer, but this risk is eliminated with intermittent fasting.

CHAPTER 7:
INTERMITTENT FASTING AND AUTOPHAGY

The word autophagy comes from a combination of the Greek word *'auto'* which means *'self,'* and the word *'phagein'* which means to eat. So, the literal translation of the word is *'to eat oneself.'* The process of autophagy is how the body eliminates all the worn-out cell machinery when there is are limited resources of energy to keep it going. It is an orderly and regulated process to recycle and degrade cellular components. Another similar process is known as apoptosis, you will also hear it referred to as programmed cell death. Once cells have been divided a certain number of times, they die automatically. The body must go through this process to maintain good health.

Think about it like this; let's imagine you've been driving the same car for 20 years, you love the car, you have awesome memories with it, and you enjoy driving it. However, the car is starting to look its age and because of how badly the parts have worn down, it's costing you a lot of money to maintain it. It's becoming more expensive to keep the car than to get rid of it, so you decide to buy a new one. This is the same thing that happens with the body, cells become junky and old, and the best course of action is to get rid of the old cells and replace them with new ones. You can also compare it to leasing a car, once the lease runs out, you've got to replace the car whether it has broken down or not. Once you have a new car, you don't need to worry about it breaking down at a time when you need it the most.

Autophagy - The Replacement of Old Cell Parts

This process also takes place at a sub-cellular level; there are times when there is no need to get a new car but to change the battery or the breaks instead. The same thing happens with the cells, instead of killing the whole cell (apoptosis), you only need to replace certain parts of the cell, this is the process of autophagy. It involves the destruction of sub-cellular organelles and the rebuilding of new ones to replace it. Organelles, old cell membranes and other cellular debris can be eliminated. This takes place through transmitting it to the lysosome which is a specialized organelle that contains enzymes to break down proteins.

The first mention of autophagy was in 1962 when researchers realized that after infusing rat liver cells with glucagon, there was an increase in lysosomes.

The term 'autophagy' was coined by the Christian de Duve, the Novel prize-winning scientist. Unused proteins and damaged sub cellular parts are labelled for elimination and then sent to the lysosomes to complete the job.

Mammalian target of rapamycin (mTOR) is one of the main regulators of autophagy. When it is dormant it supresses autophagy, and when it is active it promotes it.

Autophagy Activation

The key activator of autophagy is nutrient deprivation, glucagon is almost the opposite of the hormone insulin. When there is an insulin spike, there is a drop in glucagon; and when there is a drop in insulin, glucagon spikes. When we eat, there is an increase in insulin and a decrease in glucagon. When we don't eat (during fasting), glucagon goes up and insulin goes down. The process of autophagy is stimulated by the increase in glucagon. Research suggests that fasting causes the highest boost in autophagy.

The body experiences more benefits from fasting than just stimulating autophagy. As you have read, when autophagy is stimulated, we are getting rid of all our old cellular parts and junky proteins. At the same time, growth hormones are also stimulated when we fast which instructs our body to start producing new cells.

Before you can replenish with the new, you've got to eliminate the old which means that the destruction and the creation process are just as important as each other. Therefore, fasting helps to slow down the aging process by destroying old cells and replacing them with new ones.

Autophagy is a Very Controlled Process
The body's system carefully controls the process of autophagy. When there is a complete depletion of amino acids in mammalian cells, it is a robust indication for autophagy, but there is a lot more to the role of individual amino acids with this process. However, there is only a slight variation with plasma amino acid levels. It is believed that growth factor and amino acid signals/insulin signals merge and along the mTOR pathway.

Therefore, during autophagy, aged cell components are transformed into the amino acid components. When the body is in the beginning stages of starvation, there is an increase in amino acid levels, it is believed that the amino acids that come from autophagy are transported to the liver for gluconeogenesis. They are also turned into glucose through the tricrboxylic acid (TCA) cycle. The final step is that amino acids are changed into new proteins.

When the body fails to go through the process of autophagy, it manifests as cancer and Alzheimer's disease.

Eating turns off autophagy, proteins and insulin shut off this self-cleaning process, even a small amount of eating will do so which is why fasting is essential to gaining the full benefits associated with autophagy.

Protein Cycling - Why is it Important to Women
Protein cycling is of major importance to women because they are vulnerable to more types of cancer and their bodies hold onto more fat than men which has a negative effect on their hormones. Therefore, fasting can be extremely beneficial for women.

What is Protein Cycling?
The body is not capable of producing protein, we can only get it from food sources. Women need protein to support hormonal health and burn fat, as with men,

protein also makes women feel fuller and helps them overcome the cravings that makes it difficult for them to fast. Protein cycling involves alternating between high and low protein intake, this prevents the body from settling down and tricks it into using protein more effectively.

The reason behind consuming low amounts of protein is that when we don't eat enough, the body is forced to recycle the protein it has available and this activates autophagy. When autophagy stops, old age and disease accelerates in the body.

It is also important to mention that although you need to increase your protein intake, don't go overboard. When the body gets more protein than it needs, it goes into a state of panic. It tries to protect the body from getting poisoned by regulating every protein destroying enzyme. The average woman should consume 46 grams of protein per day; therefore, a high amount of protein would be double your normal amount. Therefore, do not consume more than 92 grams of protein per day.

One of the most effective ways for women to fast is the one meal a day fast where all your protein is consumed during your fasting window. The time that you are not eating is considered your low protein intake period. This method leads to approximately ten percent of fat reduction.

CHAPTER 8:
THE BENEFITS FOR INTERMITTENT FASTING AS AN ANTI-AGING STRATEGY

I am going to repeat some information here, but it is necessary to get a better understanding of how intermittent fasting promotes anti-aging. As you have read, when the body is starved of food, there are several metabolic changes that take place. The body uses carbohydrates as fuel; but when we are not consuming any, it gets its energy from other places. This process is referred to as 'gluconeogenesis,' it is where the body gets its glucose from sources such as amino acids.

Evidence for gluconeogenesis is found by evaluating the levels of specific metabolites in the blood such as butyrate and carnitines. Scientists have found that after fasting, these levels increase; however, they also identify several other metabolic changes such as a significant increase in the citric acid production cycle. The citric acid cycle takes place in mitochondria and its job is to release the energy that the body has stored. The increase seen in the metabolites that takes place during this process means that mitochondria has gone into overdrive.

Another discovery was the increase in pyrimidine and purine, although this increase has not been linked to fasting, the presence of these chemicals is a sign of gene expression and increased protein synthesis. This is an indication that fasting leads the cells to change the type and the quantity of proteins that they need to function.

Anti-Aging Compounds and Fasting

Elevated levels of pyrimidine and purine are signs that the levels of certain antioxidants are increasing in the body, this includes carnosine and ergothioneine. In a previous study, it was discovered that several metabolites decline as we age. These metabolites include ophthalmic acid, isoleucine and leucine. In another study by the same team of researchers, it was found that fasting led to an increase in these three metabolites which might be why fasting causes an extended lifespan in rats.

In each participant, the researchers found that there were 44 metabolites that increased during fasting, some of which had a 60-fold increase. Previously, only 14 of these metabolites were linked to fasting, but further research suggests otherwise.

Scientists believe that the increase in antioxidants may be the body's survival response. During starvation, the body experiences an increase in oxidative stress, the antioxidants produced may help protect the body against the damage that free radicals can cause.

Ketone Molecules and Youth

According to Dr. Zou, vascular aging is essential to the aging process. As we age, the vessels that support different organs become extremely sensitive making them more susceptible to damage. In an attempt to discover more about vascular aging, scientists began to evaluate the changes that takes place with senescence and how to prevent them.

Dr. Zou and his team analysed the link between vascular aging and calorie restriction. The research involved using mouse models of atherosclerosis and evaluated their aortas post-mortem where several cell culture experiments were performed. The rodents were also subjected to starvation and it was discovered that they produced the molecule beta-hydroxybutyrate which is responsible for preventing vascular aging.

Beta-hydroxybutyrate is a ketone, this molecule is produced by the liver and used as a source of energy when there is no glucose available. As I have previously mentioned, during starvation or fasting, the body produces ketones, after periods of pro-longed exercise and on when on a low-carb diet. The research also found that beta-hydroxybutyrate also promotes the multiplication and the division of cells that protect the inside of blood vessels. Cellular division is an indication of cellular youth and through endothelial cells, this compound delays vascular aging.

CHAPTER 9:
HOW TO SMOOTHLY TRANSITION TO INTERMITTENT FASTING

Change is always going to be difficult no matter what you are doing; therefore, you want to make the transition as easy as possible so that you don't lose motivation and give up before you've even started. Now that you know everything you need to know about intermittent fasting, the next step is to set goals so that you are not going on this journey blindly. When you have something specific that you are working towards, it will motivate you to continue when the going gets tough. The most effective method for setting goals is to use the SMART method:

- **S** - pecific: Define your goal in great detail, what do you hope to achieve with intermittent fasting? Saying you want to lose weight is nowhere near specific enough. Exactly how much weight do you want to lose?
- **M** - easurable: You will find it very difficult to stick to your goals if you don't monitor your progress. So, if your goal is to lose ten pounds, write that down and then weigh yourself once a week to see how you are getting along.

- **A** - chievable: Don't set yourself up for failure, setting a ridiculous goal like, *"I want to lose 50 in a week"* is never going to happen not even if you starve yourself. Neither do you want it to be too easy, the goal should be difficult enough to challenge you, but realistic enough to achieve.
- **R** - ealistic: What is your daily life like? Will it allow you to go on the type of fast you are planning?
- **T** - ime bound: Set a time limit to your goals, if not you will most likely find that you keep putting it off until you just give up altogether.

Weight Loss Goals

Excess weight is known to be a risk factor in many chronic illnesses including hypertension, cardiovascular disease and diabetes. If you've decided to start intermittent fasting to lose weight, you are on the right track because it is one of the most effective weight loss strategies. It is also important that you intensify your exercise regime and reduce your calorie intake so that you keep the weight off.

Other Health Goals

If your goals for intermittent fasting are to combat other health issues or to increase energy levels, you can measure your progress by monitoring your pain levels and the symptoms associated with your condition, as well as how much you are able to reduce the amount of medication you are taking. If you suffer from type 2 diabetes, you might set a goal of maintaining a consistent level of sugar readings for a certain period of time without any significant dips or spikes. If you suffer from hypertension, your goal might be to reduce your blood pressure reading to a certain level by a specific date.

When it comes to your energy levels, you can measure them by monitoring your ability to get the things you are struggling with now done. You can also compare how you feel first thing in the morning before you start the fast and during the fast. People with low energy levels typically feel extremely groggy in the morning and find it difficult to get going without having a coffee or an energy drink. The way you feel before going to bed is also a good indicator because when the body is healthy, your energy levels shouldn't fluctuate throughout the day. Of course, it is perfectly normal to feel tired after a hard day's work but feeling totally drained is a sign that something is wrong.

Mental Health Goals

Fasting is also an effective way to improve your mental health. Coupled with medication, research suggests that it relieves symptoms of depression and anxiety. For women who are experiencing menopausal mood swings, fasting can help balance out hormone levels so that moods are more stable. Also, when glucose levels are stabilized, you are less likely to feel the irritability associated with hunger which provides significant mental health benefits.

Mental health goals will depend on your unique situation; and there is also the chance that they will be less specific than physical health or weight loss goals. It is a bit more difficult to measure how we feel, so with your mental health goals, it might be a good idea to keep a daily journal of your emotions to help monitor how you are progressing.

Despite the fact that you are still allowed to eat, fasting is difficult, and you are going to need some help. Although IF is all about the times that you eat your meals, there are so many things you can do to prepare you for the journey and keep it fun and exciting, so you don't get bored. Here are some tips to get you started.

Share Your knowledge: It sounds like a strange way to prepare for intermittent fasting, but it works for me. In life, I have learnt that I am at my best when I'm helping others, I spent a lot of my time sharing my knowledge with my friends, family members and co-workers. When I am encouraging others, I am encouraging myself, and I like to practice what I preach so it gives me extra inspiration to make sure I stick to my fasting plan. That is one of the reasons why I decided to write this book; there is only so much talking I can do, but if I get all the knowledge out of my head and onto paper, I can help a lot more people.

Your friends and family members are going to be curious as to why you are only eating at certain times, when they ask questions, it's the perfect opportunity to tell them why. If you are anything like me, you will find that the more you share your knowledge with people, the more you will want to learn and the more you will want to put what you are learning into practice.

Download Apps: I have found Pinterest to be a great app when it comes to meal planning and healthy eating. It provides links to meal ideas, grocery lists, recipes and much more. YouTube is also really good; it can help you stay motivated by listening to other people's stories and how they overcame their struggles while intermittent fasting. The MyFitnessPal's app is another great community to join. Instead of wasting time scrolling through social media, using these apps should become your new hobby, not only will you learn a lot, but they will keep you motivated and inspired on your journey.

Food Delivery: Some people find meal planning and meal prepping doesn't fit into their lifestyles, they either don't have the time, don't like cooking, can't cook or hate shopping. If you are one of these people, there are food delivery services you can use instead. It will cost you, but if you can afford it, it will make your life a lot easier. Since there are going to be people from all over the world reading this book, I can't make suggestions as to the best food delivery services to use in your area, so Google is your best friend right now. Just make sure that you choose the healthy options.

Journaling: I find journaling very therapeutic; it might not be for everyone but give it a try and see if it works for you. As you have read, there are so many health benefits associated with intermittent fasting, so there is no doubt it will change your life for the better. You never know, one day, you might decide to share your journey with the world. Journaling will help you discover your negative triggers, measure your progress, track your weight, how you feel about food, and whatever else you decide to write about. Your first journal entry should explain why you are starting intermittent fasting and your goals.

Brush Your Teeth: We all brush our teeth before going to bed at night, but with intermittent fasting, it helps to brush your teeth after your last meal. It is a cue that tricks your brain into thinking that you've had your last meal for the day. Plus, the taste of toothpaste and mouthwash isn't going to make you want to eat again. Even though brushing your teeth earlier is nothing but a trick of the mind, it works!

Ordering at Restaurants: If you decide to go out to eat, or a friend invites you out to eat, find out what's on the menu before you get there. These days, all restaurants have menu's online; if you have set your mind on the healthy option beforehand, you are less likely to give into the temptation of eating something unhealthy. You should also bring a takeaway container, restaurants don't serve normal portions, they are two to three times the normal amount which means if you eat a full meal, you will be eating more than you should be. Split the plate in half and save the rest for another eating window.

Lunch Bag Preparation: Most people have got a job and go to work every day which can make fasting difficult. I make sure I take a lunch bag to work every day and I prepare it the night before. After dinner, after I've cleaned the kitchen, I add the following to my lunch bag:

- 2 meals
- 3-4 snacks
- 2-3 bottles of water

Even though I eat dinner at home most days, I always want to make sure I have food on standby just in case I don't get home on time. What if there's a lot of traffic, what if I've got to cover someone's shift at work? There are so many what if's that could happen, the best way to deal with them is to make sure you are prepared.

Unplanned Events: Life is never consistent, there is always a spanner in the works. However, if you are going to succeed while you are fasting, you will need to have a plan for the unplanned. As mentioned, take your lunch bag with you everywhere you go. If for whatever reason you run out of food while you are out and you've got to buy something, always have a few staple food options to hand to help you overcome the temptation to buy anything else. Always think before you eat anything.

Before you start your fast, have a serious conversation with your friends and family about your plans. Tell them not to offer you food outside your feeding window. If you have a social event planned, you can change your feeding window to allow you to eat at the event and enjoy a meal and a drink with friends and family.

Do your food shopping in bulk so you always have food to hand to accommodate any cravings and to make sure you've always got food available for your feeding window. Use small Ziploc bags, to create your own individual serving size to keep with you at all times. Buying in bulk will also save you money over the long run.

Consistent Routine: You can train your appetite by establishing a routine. Our bodies will become accustomed to our routines overtime. In general, we are hungry when we expect to be hungry and not when we are actually hungry; sometimes, this is because we need fluids or because we are bored. Also, practice makes perfect, and if fasting is a skill; the more you practice it, the better you will become.

To begin your intermittent fasting journey, start with a good routine so that you will have the stamina to endure your new lifestyle change. This means waking up, going to sleep, exercising and eating at the same times every day. You can eat your snacks at whatever time during the feeding window, but all your meals should be eaten at the same time. You should also take measurements and weigh yourself at the same time. Plan your meals the week before you go shopping, then go shopping and cook your meals on the same day.

Setbacks: There is no escape from setbacks; they are going to happen, and you've simply got to accept them, get over them and keep it moving. Setbacks might include illness, procrastination, a lack of planning, fear of missing out, no self-control, a lack of discipline and not enough knowledge about fasting.

You: You will be your biggest challenge, critic and setback during your intermittent fasting journey. Many people have issues with a lack of awareness, peer pressure, consistency, discipline, self-esteem and confidence. All of which will contribute to your inability to complete your journey.

It is important to understand that no one can do this for you, if you are going to succeed, you must do everything you can to get through it. You are responsible for your emotional well-being, there is a reason why you have chosen to start intermittent fasting, and if you want to reach your goal, you will need to stay on course. Failure is not an option!

We are all different, everyone has their reasons for doing what they do, but you should be starting this journey for YOU, not just for appearances sake, but for the ultimate happiness of your soul. Believe in yourself and know that you are your number one priority, no one and nothing matters more in this life than you, and you must be your biggest fan. Become your loudest cheerleader because no one is going to stand on the side-lines and cheer for you louder than you.

Every choice you make today will affect your tomorrow; if you don't get it right today, do better tomorrow, just don't give up. Don't make decisions based on temporary feelings or needs, think about the things you do as you are doing them and always make decisions that are going to benefit you in the long run. Think about where you want to be 30 days from now, do you want to start another diet because you thought this one didn't work? Not because it didn't but because you weren't disciplined enough to reach your goals. Wouldn't it be better to feel comfortable in your own skin, to be happy with yourself and feel confident when you put on your clothes every morning? Remember, YOU are responsible for your success!

Control Your Portions and Read Labels: Just because you are eating healthy now doesn't mean you can stuff your face. Even eating too much healthy foods can make you put on weight. To prevent this type of setback, plan and prep your meals in advance, read the labels and use portion control.

CHAPTER 10:
THE BEST AND WORST FOODS FOR SUCCESSFUL INTERMITTENT FASTING

According to Lauren Harris-Pincus, the author of '*The Protein Packed Breakfast Club*', there are no restrictions or specifications about the types of foods you should eat while intermittent fasting. However, the aim is to improve your health, a healthy diet should be a lifestyle and not something you do just to lose weight. Therefore, the key to success while intermittent fasting is to consume a well-balanced diet comprised of the following:

Cruciferous Veggies: Foods such as cauliflower, Brussels sprouts and broccoli are all high in fiber. Due to the fact that you've changed your eating pattern, it's essential that you eat fiber-rich foods to prevent constipation and keep you regular. Another advantage of fiber is that it fills you up which means you won't be as tempted to snack during your non-eating window.

Fish: Not only is fish packed with healthy proteins and fats, it' also a powerful source of vitamin D. If you are going to be eating a limited amount of food throughout the day, you want to consume foods that have a high nutritional content and fish is one of them. Also, reducing your calorie intake is known to cause brain fog and one of the many benefits of eating fish is that it's high in omega 3 which is good for the brain.

Avocado: Although avocado is extremely high in calories, the monosaturated fat in avocado is very satiating. One study found that by adding just half an avocado to your lunch will keep you full for several hours longer than if you didn't eat it.

Potatoes: According to research, potatoes are one of the most satiating foods around. Other studies have found that eating potatoes assist with weight loss. However, potato chips and French fries don't count.

Probiotics: Probiotic rich foods such as kraut, kombucha and kefir will eliminate some of the side effects associated with hunger such as constipation.

Legumes and Beans: Beans and legumes are low calorie carbohydrates that will provide you with more than enough fuel to keep you going throughout the day. Foods such as lentils, peas, black beans and chickpeas help you lose weight without restricting your calorie intake.

Berries: Strawberries and blueberries are high in flavonoids and studies have found that they help to reduce body mass index (BMI) over time. Strawberries are also a rich source of vitamin C which boosts the immune system. You can get 100 percent of your daily value in one cup of strawberries.

Eggs: There are six grams of protein in one large egg and protein is essential for building muscle and keeping full. One study discovered that men who ate an egg for breakfast instead of a bagel were not as hungry throughout the day.

Whole Grains: Whole grains are rich in protein and fiber which means that you don't need to eat much of them to get full. Additionally, one study found that consuming whole grains instead of refined grains boosts the metabolism.

Nuts: They may contain more calories than any other snacks, but nuts are packed full of good fats and studies have found that the polyunsaturated fat in walnuts can transform the physiological markers for satiety and hunger.

Water: Last but not least, water! Even though you don't eat water, whether you are intermittent fasting or not, you need to stay hydrated because the health of every major organ in your body depends on it. You will often hear experts state that adults should drink 2 liters of water per day; however, for some people, that might be too much. You will know when you've drank enough water if your urine is pale yellow in colour. When your urine is dark yellow, it is a sign that you are dehydrated which causes light-headedness, fatigue and headaches. On the other hand, you can also drink too much water, and clear, colorless urine is an indication of this. If you don't enjoy drinking plain water, add a squeeze of lemon, cucumber slices or mint leaves to it.

Foods to Stay Away from While Intermittent Fasting

Whether you are intermittent fasting or not, there are some foods that you should cut out of your diet altogether. However, when it comes to IF, it is also important to mention that if your goal is to lose weight, there is no point consuming an entire days' worth of food during your eating window because your weight will either remain the same or you will put on weight if you are consuming too many calories. Here are some of the foods you should eliminate from your diet while intermittent fasting.

Pizzas: Everyone loves pizza; unfortunately, the majority of commercial pizzas are made out of very unhealthy ingredients such as processed meat and refined dough. They are also high in calories which is a double negative if you are trying to lose weight. This doesn't mean you can't make your own pizza, just make a healthy alternative with wholesome ingredients.

Fruit Juices: We have been deceived into believing that fruit juices are good for us because they contain fruit. But what the advertisements fail to tell us is that they are packed with unhealthy refined sugar. Although they contain healthy ingredients such as vitamin C and antioxidants, some fruit juices contain the same amount of sugar as fizzy drinks such as Pepsi or Coke; and in some cases, even more.

White Bread: Refined wheat contains little to no essential nutrients and because it has been stripped of wholegrains, white bread is low in fiber; and when eaten, causes a spike in blood sugar. Whole grain and Ezekiel bread are healthy alternatives.

Breakfast Cereals: Sweetened breakfast cereals are popular among children, they are processed cereal grains, such as corn, rice, oats and wheat. To give them additional flavor, the grains are flaked, rolled, pulped, shredded or roasted and are typically high in sugar. Healthy alternatives are breakfast cereals that are low in added sugar and high in fiber.

Cakes, Cookies and Pastries: These snacks are typically made with refined wheat flour, refined sugar and added fats. Some of them also contain shortening which is high in trans fats. Unfortunately, these tasty treats are high in calories, high in preservatives and contain no essential nutrients.

Agave Nectar: This is another deceptive unhealthy ingredient; however, it is exceptionally high in fructose and it is extremely refined. In fact, agave nectar contains more fructose than any other sweetener. High-fructose corn syrup contains 55% fructose, table sugar contains around 50% fructose and agave nectar is made up of 85% fructose. Erythritol and Stevia are healthy, calorie free and natural alternatives.

Low-Carb Junk Foods: Again, there are many foods that are touted as healthy, but they are far from it.

Foods such as low-carb meal replacements and candy bars are packed with additives and highly processed. If you want to stop eating so many carbs, eat foods that are naturally low in carbs such as leafy greens, seafood and eggs.

Ice Cream: Everyone loves ice-cream, but it's full of sugar. My advice is that you make your own healthy version.

There are so many foods that are good and bad for you, that I could write an entire book on the subject. My advice to you is to read food labels to check for sugar content and ingredients that are difficult to read. That is typically an indicator that it is highly processed.

CHAPTER 11:
HOW TO STAY MOTIVATED WHILE INTERMITTENT FASTING

We all know what motivation feels like. It's a high, an energy that makes us enjoy our life, and the things we're doing. Motivation fuels us to work harder, to get more done, to achieve more. You were probably motivated to buy this book after reading or watching a success story about intermittent fasting. Highly motivated people are more successful. Unfortunately, motivation doesn't last very long. The motivation you feel often disappears after a few days, maybe even a few hours. We've all had the experiences of being highly motivated to become more active and fit: we join a gym, maybe buy workout clothes and an exercise DVD. But then after a few days, we lose the motivation: it just disappears into thin air.

The good news is, that motivation can be created, and called upon at will. It just takes some practice. There are some who say, why bother with motivation when it never lasts very long? Yes, it's true that motivation doesn't last very long – but neither does bathing, nor eating. That's why we do those things every day! Just like bathing, eating and other essential life activities, motivation needs to be practiced regularly. Try to make it a part of your daily routine to motivate yourself and you will see your life improving by leaps and bounds. Here are three things you can do to increase your motivation while intermittent fasting.

Have a Vision Board: The easiest way to motivate yourself is to see what you want. Instead of just imagining things, make it easy to be close to what you want by seeing exactly what you want. A vision board has images of the thing that you'd like in your life. So, whatever your intermittent fasting goals are, whether it's to lose weight, gain more energy, or improve your health, find visual images of these goals and create a vision board out of them.

A vision board can be a physical board with printed photos and art posted on it. Or you can use software apps to create a digital vision board. I like to have things that inspire me on my desktop background; this way, when I need motivation, all I have to do is glance at my background.

Keep motivating images handy, so that whenever you need a quick dose of motivation, you can look at your vision board. For instance, I like to look at motivating exercise quotes and photos before I exercise – this ensures that I exercise harder.

Complete an Act of Power: Always start your day with an act of power. An action that nobody's forcing you to do, that you choose to do of your own volition which makes life better. An act of power should be short and easy to complete. US Army Seals always start their day with an act of power: the act of making their beds. Making your bed is a great act of power because it accomplishes many things. It establishes neatness and order in your bedroom, it signals the end of time spent in bed, and completes your first task of the day. An act of power first thing in the morning establishes that you are in control. You're the one driving your life to success. You have the power and the ability to get things done.

Have a Morning Routine: As well as having an act of power, a great way to start your day is with a positive energizing morning routine. Your morning routine should be customized to your lifestyle, and help you get in the right mood for the day.

Have Long and Short-Term Goals: One of the main reasons why people fail at anything in life is they fail to have short term goals. If you want to lose 100 lbs. through intermittent fasting, there is a high chance you will give up within a week or two of making the commitment because your brain can't handle such high numbers. As you have read, motivation doesn't last so for the idea of losing that much weight is only going to sound good for as long as your motivation lasts. Once you run out of motivation, you will start making excuses as to why you need to eat outside of your eating window, and before you know it, you have abandoned the goal.

The easiest way to achieve your long-term goals is to break them down into short term goals. So instead of saying you want to lose 100 lbs., say you want to lose 2 lbs. per week. Two is a small number, when you look at it on your vision board it won't fill you with dread in the same way that 100 will. By aiming to lose 2 lbs. per week, you will lose the full 100 lbs. within 12 months.

Surround Yourself with Positive People: Some people are going to find what you are doing strange, especially your former eating partners. I am in no way knocking fat people, I am just using this as an example, so please don't get offended. Fat people usually have fat friends, and when one of them wants to lose weight and the rest are not ready, they adopt a crab in the bucket mentality and try and keep the person who wants to lose weight on the same level. No matter whether you want to start intermittent fasting to lose weight, or to get healthier, if your immediate social circle is not cheering you on, you will need to keep them at arm's length, or they will totally derail your efforts. Join a Facebook group with other like-minded people who are on the same journey as you and will encourage you as you go on your way.

CHAPTER 12:
EXERCISE RECOMMENDATIONS
WHILE INTERMITTENT FASTING

There are a lot of debates surrounding whether you should exercise during intermittent fasting. I am not here to add to the argument, all I know is that I exercise while fasting and I have never had a problem. What I can say is that there are a number of strategies you can implement to make your work out more effective.

It's All About Timing

Registered dietician Christopher Shuff states that you should think about three things before starting an exercise routine while fasting. Whether you should exercise during your eating window, before or after it.

LeanGains 16:8 protocol is a popular method of intermittent fasting, and as mentioned it involves eating within an 8-hour window and then fasting for 16 hours. Some people perform well exercising on an empty stomach, and some people perform better exercising after they have eaten. However, Shuff states that if you want to take advantage of performance and recovery, working out during the eating window is best. This way, your body can tap into glycogen stores to fuel your workout.

Think About Your Macros

Certified personal trainer Lynda Lippin argues that you should pay attention to the macronutrients you are consuming the day before you exercise and when you eat afterwards. For example, workouts for strength typically need more carbohydrates the day of, and high intensity interval training/cardio can be done when you have eaten less carbohydrates.

Eat the Right Meals

Dr Niket Sonpal says the best solution for combining exercise and intermittent fasting is to time your workouts during your eating window so that you have high levels of nutrition in your system. If you lift heavy weights, it's important to consume a lot of protein after working out to assist with the regeneration process. Additionally, any strength training should be followed up with around 20 grams of protein and carbohydrates 30 minutes after your workout.

Stay Hydrated

Fasting does not mean you should stop drinking water, make sure you get enough water throughout the day to ensure that you stay hydrated.

Electrolytes

Coconut water is a good low-calorie hydration source; sports drinks such as Gatorade are high in sugar so you should avoid drinking them often.

Duration and Intensity

If you push yourself too hard and you start feeling light-headed and dizzy, take a break. It's important to listen to your body.

The Type of Fast

Stick to low-intensity workouts such as gentle Pilates, restorative yoga and walking if you are doing a 24-hour fast. However, if you are doing the 16:8 fast, you can stick to your normal workout routine because you are not going the entire day without food.

Listen to Your Body

The most important advice to take into consideration when it comes to exercising during intermittent fasting is to listen to your body. If you start feeling dizzy or weak, your blood sugar is probably low, or you are dehydrated. To recover, have a carbohydrate-electrolyte drink straight away and then eat a well-balanced meal.

Although intermittent fasting and exercise might

work for some people, it might not work for others. Therefore, give it a try and see how you feel; if your body doesn't agree, stop.

CHAPTER 13:
WEIGHT LOSS RECIPES TO SUPERCHARGE YOUR JOURNEY

BREAKFAST RECIPES

Peanut Butter and Jelly Overnight Oats

Preparation Time: 5 Minutes (8 hours in the fridge)/Servings: 1 Serving

Nutritional Value: Fat: 28 grams/Fiber: 9 grams/Protein: 20 grams/Calories: 455

Ingredients

- ¼ cup of rolled oats, fast cooking
- ½ a cup of 2% milk
- 3 tablespoons of creamy peanut butter
- ¼ cup of crushed raspberries
- 3 tablespoons of whole raspberries

Directions

1. Combine the mashed raspberries, peanut butter, milk and oats in a medium bowl and mix together thoroughly.
2. Put a lid over the bowl and let it sit in the fridge overnight.
3. In the morning, remove the cover, top with the whole raspberries and serve.

Tofu Turmeric Scramble

Preparation Time: 15 Minutes/Servings: 1 Serving

Nutritional Value: Fat: 33 grams/Fiber: 8 grams/Protein: 21 grams/Calories: 431

Ingredients

- 1 portobello mushroom
- A handful of cherry tomatoes
- 1 tablespoon of olive oil and some extra for brushing
- Salt and pepper
- ½ a block of firm tofu
- ¼ teaspoon of ground turmeric
- 1 pinch of garlic powder
- ½ a thinly sliced avocado

Directions

1. Prepare the oven by heating it to 400 degrees F.
2. Arrange the cherry tomatoes and the portobello mushroom on a baking sheet, coat them with oil and then season with salt and pepper. Roast for approximately 10 minutes until they become tender.

3. Combine the tofu, garlic powder, turmeric
   and a pinch of salt in a medium bowl and use
   a fork to mash the ingredients together.

4. Heat the olive oil in a frying pan over medium
   heat, add the tofu mixture, stir occasionally
   and cook until it becomes firm like egg. This
   should take about 3 minutes.

5. Spoon the tofu onto a plate, add the cherry
   tomatoes and the avocado and serve.

Green Smoothie

Preparation Time: 5 Minutes/Servings: 1 Serving

Nutritional Value: Fat: 1.3 grams/Fiber: 4.5 grams/Protein: 4.3 grams/Calories: 184

Ingredients

- 1 tablespoon of chia seeds
- 1 cup of chard, kale or spinach
- 1 small handful of blueberries
- 1 cup of coconut milk
- 1 avocado

Directions

1. Combine all the ingredients together into a food processor and blend until smooth.
2. Pour into a cup and serve.

Yogurt and Banana Crunch

Preparation Time: 5 Minutes/Servings: 1 Serving

Nutritional Value: Fat: 4.1 grams/Fiber: 12.8 grams/Protein: 10.2 grams/Calories: 328.5

Ingredients

- 12 ounces of fat free Greek yogurt
- 1 banana, peeled and sliced
- ½ an ounce of mixed seeds or mixed nuts of your choice

Directions

- Pour the Greek yogurt into two bowls.
- Top with the banana.
- Sprinkle the seeds or the nuts over the top.

Tomato and Bacon Poached Eggs

Preparation Time: 20 Minutes/Servings: 2 Servings

Nutritional Value: Fat: 25 grams/Fiber: 0 grams/Protein: 22 grams/Calories: 458

Ingredients

- 2 large eggs
- 2 large tomatoes sliced in half
- 4 strips of low-sodium, low-fat bacon
- Salt
- Black pepper

Directions

1. Prepare the grill by pre-heating it to the highest setting.
2. Line foil over a grill pan and arrange the halved tomatoes onto it.
3. Sprinkle the black pepper over the tomatoes.
4. Grill the tomatoes for around 3 minutes.
5. Add the bacon to the grill and continue to grill for a further two minutes until the bacon turns light brown on both sides.
6. Boil water in a large saucepan.
7. Crack the eggs into two separate bowls and make sure the yolks are kept intact.

8. Turn the heat down until the water begins to simmer gently.

9. Gently slide the eggs into the simmering water and leave it to cook for about three minutes.

10. You will know it is cooked when the whites are set but the yolks are runny.

11. Use a spoon to scoop the poached eggs out of the water and place them onto two plates.

12. Arrange the cooked tomatoes and the bacon onto the plates, sprinkle with salt and pepper before serving.

Garlic and Mushroom Frittata

Preparation Time: 20 Minutes/Servings: 2 Servings

Nutritional Value: Fat: 14 grams/Fiber: 2.5 grams/Protein: 14 grams/Calories: 243

Ingredients

- 4 large eggs
- 1 clove of crushed garlic
- 1 tablespoon of thinly sliced chives
- 9 ounces of sliced chestnut mushrooms
- Black pepper
- Cooking spray

Directions

1. Spray a frying pan with cooking spray and heat it over a medium temperature.
2. Add the mushrooms and cook until they turn golden brown in colour.
3. Turn the temperature to high and add the crushed garlic and chives until cooked. Sprinkle with pepper and stir to combine.
4. Preheat the grill on the highest temperature.
5. Whisk the eggs in a small bowl and pour them over the mushroom mixture.

6. Cook for about 5 minutes until the bottom has
   set.
7. Place the frying pan in the grill and cook for a
   further five minutes until the eggs are full set.
8. Remove from the grill, divide onto plates and
   serve.

Pear and Cinnamon Porridge

Preparation Time: 30 Minutes/Servings: 2 Serving

Nutritional Value: Fat: 8 grams/Fiber: 6 grams/Protein: 7.5 grams/Calories: 267

Ingredients

- 2.5 ounces of oats
- ¼ teaspoon of ground cinnamon plus extra for sprinkling
- 10 ounces of semi skimmed milk
- 1 ripened pear
- 1 lemon wedge

Directions

1. Combine the oats, cinnamon and milk in a non-stick saucepan on a low to medium temperature for approximately 5 minutes. Keep stirring until the oats turn into a creamy consistency.
2. Pour the oats into bowls, grate the pear over and squeeze the lemon wedge over the top. Sprinkle with extra cinnamon and serve.

Berries with Yogurt

Preparation Time: 5 Minutes/Servings: 2 Serving

Nutritional Value: Fat: 3 grams/Fiber: 3 grams/Protein: 14 grams/Calories: 220

Ingredients

- 6 ounces of fresh or frozen berries of your choice
- 12 ounces of fat-free Greek yogurt
- 10 ounces of toasted almond flakes or almond slivers

Preparation

1. Pour a layer of yogurt into each bowl.
2. Sprinkle a layer of berries over the top.
3. Pour a layer of yogurt over the top.
4. Sprinkle a layer of berries over the top.
5. Sprinkle the almonds over the top and serve.

Mushroom Delight

Preparation Time: 25 Minutes/Servings: 1 Serving

Nutritional Value: Fat: 23 grams/Fiber: 0.9 grams/Protein: 18 grams/Calories: 230

Ingredients

- 10 ounces of chopped portobello mushrooms
- 3 ounces of chopped green beans
- 2 ounces of grated zucchini
- 1 spring onion
- 2 large eggs
- 1 clove of minced garlic
- 5 ounces of mustard
- 5 ounces of grated cheese

Directions

1. Combine all the mushrooms, green beans, zucchini, onion, eggs, minced garlic and mustard into a frying pan. Cook for 5 to 10 minutes over a medium temperature.
2. Break the eggs over the mixture and leave the mixture to cook for an additional two minutes until the egg whites are firm.
3. Scoop the mushroom delight onto plates, sprinkle with grated cheese and serve.

Colourful Berry and Banana Smoothie

Preparation Time: 5 Minutes/Servings: 1 Serving

Nutritional Value: Fat: 1.7 grams/Fiber: 2.8 grams/Protein: 5.5 grams/Calories: 161

Ingredients

- 1 handful of blueberries
- 1 handful of raspberries
- 1 ripe banana
- Half a cup of semi-skimmed milk

Directions

1. Combine all the ingredients into a food processor and blend until smooth.
2. Pour into a glass and serve.

Hot Mixed Grain Cereal

Preparation Time: 35 Minutes/Serves: 4 Servings

Nutritional Value: Fat: 2 grams/Fiber: 3 grams/Protein: 10 grams/Calories: 210

Ingredients

- ½ a teaspoon of ground cinnamon
- 6 tablespoons of couscous, plain and uncooked
- 1 cup of apple, sliced and peeled
- 2 tablespoons of buckwheat, uncooked
- 2 tablespoons of bulgur, uncooked
- ¼ cups of rice milk, vanilla
- 2 ¼ cups of water

Directions

1. Heat the milk and water over medium-high heat in a medium sized saucepan and let the ingredients boil.
2. Add the buckwheat, bulgur and apple.
3. Turn the heat down to low and leave the ingredients to simmer, stir occasionally until the bulgur becomes tender. This should take around 25 minutes.

4. Take the saucepan off the cooker, add the
    cinnamon and the couscous and stir to
    combine.
5. Put the lid onto the saucepan and leave it to
    rest of 10 minutes before fluffing with a fork.
6. Divide into bowls and serve

Egg in the Hole

Preparation time: 10 Minutes/Serves: 2 Servings

Nutritional Value: Fat: 10.1 grams/Fiber: 1.8 grams/Protein: 9.1 grams/Calories: 181.2

Ingredients

- Freshly ground black pepper
- A pinch of cayenne pepper
- 2 tablespoons of fresh, chopped chives
- 2 eggs
- ¼ cup of unsalted butter
- 2 slices of Italian bread, ½ an inch thick

Directions

1. Use a small glass or a cookie cutter to cut a 2-inch round out of the middle of each piece of bread.
2. Melt the butter over medium temperature in a large non-stick frying pan.
3. Put the bread into the frying pan and toast it for 30 seconds on each side.
4. Break the eggs into the cut-out holes in the middle of the bread and cook for approximately 2 minutes. Make sure the eggs

are set and the bread has turned a golden
brown in colour.

5. Top with the black pepper, cayenne pepper
   and chives.
6. Repeat with the other slice of bread, arrange
   onto plates and serve.

Baked Pancake

Preparation Time: 35 Minutes/Serves: 2 Servings

Nutritional Value: Fat: 10.1 grams/Fiber: 2.4 grams/Protein: 10.6 grams/Calories: 208.7

Ingredients

- Cooking spray to grease the skillet
- A pinch of ground nutmeg
- 4 a teaspoon of ground cinnamon
- ½ a cup of all-purpose flour
- ½ a cup of rice milk, unsweetened
- 2 eggs

Directions

1. Prepare the oven by heating it to 450 degrees F.
2. Whisk together the rice milk and eggs in a medium sized bowl.
3. Add the nutmeg, cinnamon and flour and continue to stir until everything is combined but still a bit lumpy.
4. Spray an oven-proof frying pan with cooking spray and heat it in the oven for 5 minutes.
5. Pour the batter into the frying pan and put it back into the oven to bake for 20 minutes. The

pancake is cooked when its crispy around the edges and puffed up.

6. Remove from the oven, transfer onto plates and serve.

French Toast Stuffed with Cream Cheese and Strawberries

Preparation Time: 1 Hour 5 Minutes/Serves: 4 Servings

Nutritional Value: Fat: 22.2 grams/Fiber: 4.6 grams/Protein: 15.7 grams/Calories: 499

Ingredients

- ¼ teaspoon of ground cinnamon
- 1 tablespoon of granulated sugar
- 1 teaspoon of pure vanilla extract
- ½ a cup of rice milk, unsweetened
- 8 slices of thick white bread
- 4 tablespoons of strawberry jam
- ½ a cup of plain cream cheese
- Cooking spray to grease the baking dish
-

Directions

1. Spray the baking dish with cooking spray and put it to one side.
2. Combine the jam and cheese in a small bowl and mix together thoroughly.
3. Spread 3 tablespoons of the cream mixture over 4 slices of bread and put the other 4 slices of bread over the top to make sandwiches.

4. Whisk the vanilla, eggs and milk together in a small bowl until the ingredients become smooth.
5. Dip the sandwiches into the egg mixture and arrange them into the baking dish.
6. Pour the rest of the egg mixture on top of the sandwiches and sprinkle cinnamon and sugar over the top.
7. Place foil over the baking dish and leave them it in the fridge overnight.
8. The next day, prepare the oven by heating it to 350 degrees F.
9. Remove the baking tray from the fridge and bake the French toast for 1 hour.
10. Take the foil off the baking tray and bake until the toast turns into a golden brown colour. This should take about five minutes.
11. Once cooked, remove from the oven, arrange onto plates and serve.

Scrambled Cheesy Eggs with Fresh Herbs

Preparation Time: 25 Minutes/Serves: 4 Servings

Nutritional Value: Fat: 8.1 grams/Fiber: 0 grams/Protein: 6.9 grams/Calories: 107

Ingredients

- Freshly ground black pepper
- 2 tablespoons of unsalted butter
- 1 tablespoon of fresh tarragon
- 1 tablespoon of finely chopped scallion – the green part only
- ¼ cup of rice milk, unsweetened
- ½ a cup of cream cheese, room temperature
- 2 egg whites, room temperature
- 3 eggs, room temperature
-

Directions

1. Combine the tarragon, scallions, rice milk, cream cheese, egg whites and eggs in a medium bowl and whisk together thoroughly.
2. Heat the butter in a large frying pan over medium-high heat.
3. Add the egg mixture and stir until it turns into a scramble. Season with salt and pepper.
4. Divide onto plates and serve.

Pineapple and Blueberry Smoothie

Preparation Time: 15 Minutes/Serves: 2 Servings

Nutritional Value: Fat: 3.4 grams/Fiber: 1.3 grams/Protein: 1.3 grams/Calories: 230

Ingredients

- ½ a cup of water
- ½ an apple
- ½ a cup of English cucumber
- ½ a cup of pineapple chunks
- 1 cup of frozen blueberries
-

Directions

1. Combine all the ingredients into a food processor and blend until smooth.
2. Pour into glasses and serve.

Pepper and Tarragon Pasta Salad

Preparation Time: 45 Minutes/Serves: 4 Servings

Nutritional Value: Fat: 23 grams/Fiber: 2 grams/Protein: 16 grams/Calories: 390

Ingredients

- 1 tablespoon of dried tarragon
- 2 tablespoons of extra virgin olive oil
- 1 teaspoon of black pepper
- ¼ finely sliced red onion
- ½ a finely diced cucumber
- 1 finely sliced red bell pepper
- 2 cups of white pasta

Directions

1. Boil a large saucepan of water and cook the pasta according to the directions on the packet.
2. Once cooked, drain the water from the pasta and leave it to cool down.
3. Add the rest of the ingredients to the pasta and toss to combine.
4. Divide onto plates and serve.

Apple and Brie Salad

Preparation Time: 5 Minutes/Serves: 2 Servings

Nutritional Value: Fat: 36.1 grams/Fiber: 8.4 grams/Protein: 11.9 grams/Calories: 493

Ingredients

- ½ a peeled and apple, cored and diced
- ½ a cup of sliced brie
- 1 teaspoon of white wine vinegar
- 1 cup of watercress

Directions

1. Put the watercress into a medium sized bowl and toss with vinegar.
2. Add the apple and brie and toss to combine.
3. Serve with crackers or Melba toast.

Curried Couscous and Baked Salmon

Preparation Time: 25 Minutes/Serves: 2 Servings

Nutritional Value: Fat: 13 grams/Fiber: 3 grams/Protein: 4 grams/Calories: 230

Ingredients

- 1 tablespoon of chili powder
- 1 tablespoon of curry powder
- 2 cups of water
- 1 cup of chicken stock
- 2 cloves of minced garlic
- 1 diced green onion
- 2 tablespoons of extra virgin olive oil
- 2 salmon steaks
- Salt and black pepper
- The juice of 1 lemon

Directions for the Couscous

1. Heat the olive oil in a large saucepan over a medium temperature.
2. Add the garlic, onions and sauté until they become soft, this should take around 2 minutes.
3. Add the couscous and stir until it becomes slightly toasted.

4. Add the water, the chicken stock, increase the heat to high and once it starts to boil reduce the heat to low.
5. Add the chili powder and the curry.
6. Put a lid over the saucepan and leave the ingredients to simmer until the couscous has soaked up the majority of the liquid. This should take around 20 minutes.
7. Stir through the couscous with a fork

Directions for the Salmon
1. Heat the oven to 350 degrees F.
2. Line a baking tray with foil.
3. In a small bowl, combine the lemon juice and salt and pepper.
4. Arrange the salmon on the baking tray and brush it with the lemon mixture.
5. Bake the salmon for 20 minutes until it flakes when poked with a fork.
6. Once cooked, remove from the oven and serve with the couscous.

Cauliflower and Onion Curried Soup

Preparation Time: 50 Minutes/Serves: 4 Servings

Nutritional Value: Fat: 7.1 grams/Fiber: 5.8 grams/Protein: 5.5 grams/Calories: 131.3

Ingredients

- 1 cup of low-fat coconut milk
- 3 cups of water
- 1 cup of chicken broth
- 1 teaspoon of turmeric
- 1 teaspoon of cumin
- 3 sticks of chopped celery
- ½ a chopped cauliflower
- 4 cloves of minced garlic
- 1 chopped onion
- 2 tablespoons of coconut oil

Directions

1. In a large saucepan, heat the oil over medium to high heat.
2. Add the cauliflower, garlic and onions leave them to steam for 5 to 10 minutes.
3. Add the spices and celery and cook for a further 5 minutes.
4. Add the water and the stock and once the ingredients start to boil, turn the heat down

and simmer until the celery is soft. This
should take approximately 15-20 minutes.

5. Take the saucepan from the fire and allow the
soup to cool down.

6. Pour the soup into a food processor blend
until smooth.

7. Pour the soup back into the saucepan and
heat.

8. Add the coconut oil and stir to combine.

9. Sprinkle with black pepper, spoon into bowls
and serve.

Pitta Pizza with BBQ Chicken

Preparation Time: 30 Minutes/Serves: 2 Servings

Nutritional Value: Fat: 14 grams/Fiber: 1.3 grams/Protein: 20 grams/Calories: 356

Ingredients

- 2 pieces of pita bread
- ⅛ teaspoon of garlic powder
- 4 ounces of cooked chicken
- 2 tablespoons of feta cheese, crumbled
- ¼ cup of purple onion
- 3 tablespoons of barbeque sauce, low sodium
- Cooking spray

Directions

1. Prepare the oven by heating it to 350 degrees F.
2. Grease a baking tray with the cooking spray and arrange the pita bread onto it.
3. Sprinkle the onion over the pitas.
4. Spread the chicken over the top.
5. Sprinkle the feta cheese over the top.
6. Sprinkle the garlic powder over the top.
7. Bake the pitas for 15 minutes.
8. Once cooked, remove from the oven and serve.

Heart-Warming Vegetable Soup

Preparation Time: 45 Minutes/Servings: 2 Serving

Nutritional Value: Fat: 3.8 grams/Fiber: 3.4 grams/Protein: 5.8 grams/Calories: 159

Ingredients

- 1 sliced onion
- 2 cloves of sliced garlic
- 2 carrots cut into chunks
- 1 can of chopped tomatoes
- 2 celery sticks, sliced
- 1 cube of vegetable stock
- 1 can of lima beans rinsed and drained
- 4 ounces of sliced spring greens
- Salt and pepper
- Cooking spray
- 2 slices of crispy French bread

Directions

1. Spray a large saucepan with cooking oil and heat over a medium temperature.
2. Add the garlic, onion, celery and carrots and cook for 10 minutes until the ingredients become soft.

3. Add the chopped tomatoes to the pan as well as 26 ounces of water.
4. Add the salt and pepper to taste and stir to combine.
5. Turn the heat up to high until it starts to boil and then reduce the heat to low.
6. Leave the ingredients to simmer for 20 minutes.
7. Add the lima beans, spring greens and leave the soup to simmer for 5 minutes.
8. Spoon the mixture into bowls and serve with the French bread.

Chili and Coriander Fish Parcel

Preparation Time: 2 Hours Servings: 1 Serving

Nutritional Value: Fat: 7.1 grams/Fiber: 0.5 grams/Protein: 15 grams/Calories: 124

Ingredients

- 4 ounces of haddock or cod fillet
- 2 teaspoons of lemon juice
- 1 tablespoon of coriander leaves
- 1 clove of garlic, chopped
- 1 green chilli, seeds removed and chopped
- ¼ teaspoon of sugar
- 2 teaspoons of Greek yogurt
- 3 ounces of steamed snow peas

Directions

1. Put the fish fillet in bowl and squeeze the lemon over the top.
2. Cover the dish with foil and put it into the fridge to marinate for 20 minutes.
3. In a food processor, combine the garlic, green chili and coriander and blend to combine until the ingredients turn into a paste.

4. Add the Greek yogurt and the sugar and
    continue to blend.
5. Remove the fish from the oven and lay it on a
    sheet of foil.
6. Spread the paste over the fish and fold the foil
    over it to create a parcel. Make sure the ends
    are sealed and put it back in the fridge to
    marinate for an hour.
7. Preheat the oven to 400 degrees F, place the
    parcelled fish onto a baking tray and bake for
    15 minutes.
8. Steam the snow peas while the fish is baking.
9. Once cooked, remove the fish from the oven,
    arrange onto a plate and serve with the snow
    peas.

Tomato and Garlic Shrimp

Preparation Time: 20 Minutes/Servings: 1 Serving

Nutritional Value: Fat: 14.1 grams/Fiber: 1.1 grams/Protein: 7.9 grams/Calories: 213.9

Ingredients

- 6 ounces of steamed green beans
- Black pepper
- 3 tablespoons of chopped parsley leaves
- 9 ounces of cooked, peeled and deveined jumbo shrimp
- The juice of ½ a lemon
- 5 ounces of cherry tomatoes cut into halves
- 1 chopped red chilli
- 2 cloves of garlic sliced
- 1 tablespoon of cooking oil

Directions

1. Heat the cooking oil in a frying pan over a medium temperature.
2. Add the chili and garlic and cook for 5 minutes.
3. Add the cherry tomatoes and the lemon juice and cook for a further 2 minutes until the tomatoes become soft.

4. Add the shrimp and cook for another 3 minutes.
5. Take the frying pan off the cooker, add the parsley and season with black pepper.
6. Spoon onto plates and serve with the steamed green beans.

Stuffed Mushrooms

Preparation Time: 25 Minutes/Servings: 1 Serving

Nutritional Value: Fat: 3 grams/Fiber: 1 gram/Protein: 4 grams/Calories: 50

Ingredients

- 3 portobello mushrooms
- 4 ounces of low-fat ricotta cheese
- 1.5 ounces of low-fat grated cheddar cheese
- 1 ounce of diced ham
- ¼ cup of chopped fresh parsley
- 1 ounce of diced red peppers

Directions

1. Preheat the oven to 350 degrees F.
2. Remove the stems from the mushrooms and dice them.
3. Line a baking tray with foil and arrange the mushroom caps on it.
4. In a bowl, combine the diced mushroom stems, ricotta cheese, parsley, peppers and ham.
5. Spoon the mixture into the mushroom caps.
6. Sprinkle the grated cheddar cheese over the top.
7. Bake the mushrooms for 20 minutes.
8. Remove from the oven and serve.

Rice Cake Caprese

Preparation Time: 10 Minutes/Servings: 1 Serving

Nutritional Value: Fat: 28 grams/Fiber: 3 grams/Protein: 23 grams/Calories: 570

Ingredients

- 1 rice cake
- 4 cherry tomatoes sliced in halves
- ½ a teaspoon of basil leaves
- ½ a teaspoon of garlic
- 1 tablespoon of low-fat cottage cheese

Directions

1. Combine the basil and garlic in a food processor.
2. Spread the cottage cheese over the rice cake.
3. Arrange the cherry tomatoes over the top.
4. Spoon the basil and garlic mixture over top and serve.

Tuna Pesto Salad

Preparation Time: 10 Minutes/Servings: 1 Serving

*Nutritional Value: Fat: 16.3 grams/Fiber: 9.1
grams/Protein: 33 grams/Calories: 539.2*

Ingredients for the Tuna

- One 4 ounce can of tuna in oil
- 1 tablespoon of mayonnaise
- 1 tablespoon of Greek yogurt
- 1 tablespoon of pesto
- 1 tablespoons of lemon juice
- A pinch of sea salt

Ingredients for the Salad

- 4 iceberg lettuce leaves shredded
- 1 sliced tomato
- ½ a sliced cucumber
- ¼ sliced avocado

Ingredients for the Dressing

1. 1 tablespoon of olive oil
2. ½ a tablespoon of apple cider vinegar
3. Salt and pepper

Directions

1. To make the tuna combine all the ingredients together in a small bowl and combine with fork to smash the tuna.
2. To make the dressing, combine all the ingredients into a sealed container and shake to combine.
3. Arrange the lettuce, cucumber and tomato onto a plate.
4. Spoon the tuna over the top, arrange the avocado slices over the top.
5. Drizzle with the dressing and serve.

Salmon and Tabbouleh Bowl

Preparation Time: 25 Minutes/Servings: 2 Serving

Nutritional Value: Fat: 45.2 grams/Fiber: 4.3 grams/Protein: 42.8 grams/Calories: 629

Ingredients for the Salmon
- Two 10-ounce salmon fillets
- Salt and pepper
- 1 tablespoon of olive oil
- 9 ounces of cauliflower
- ½ a cup of shredded red cabbage
- ¼ cup of chopped sugar snap peas
- ⅓ cup of chopped red pepper
- ¼ diced red onion
- ¼ cup of fresh parsley, chopped
- 2 tablespoons of chopped mint
- ½ a cup of crumbled feta cheese
- 3 tablespoons of olive oil
- 2 teaspoons of fresh lemon juice

Ingredients for the Dressing
- 1 tablespoon of Greek yogurt
- 1 tablespoon of chopped basil
- 1 teaspoon of lemon juice
- Salt and black pepper

Directions

1. Prepare the oven by preheating it to 350 degrees F.
2. Line a baking sheet with foil.
3. Season the salmon with 1 teaspoon of olive oil and salt and pepper.
4. Arrange the salmon with the skin facing up onto the baking tray and cook for 25 minutes.
5. Pulse the cauliflower in a food processor until it turns into a rice like consistency.
6. Put the cauliflower in a microwave safe bowl and cook in the microwave for 4 minutes. There is no need to add water because the cauliflower contains water.
7. Once cooked, remove the cauliflower from the microwave and fluff with a fork.
8. Combine the chopped herbs, red pepper, red onion, sugar snap peas and red cabbage in a bowl and toss to combine.
9. In another bowl, combine 2 teaspoons of olive oil, lemon juice, salt and pepper and whisk together thoroughly.
10. Add the olive oil mixture and half of the feta cheese mixture to the cauliflower rice and toss to combine.
11. In a small bowl, combine the ingredients for the dressing and mix together thoroughly.

12. Spoon the tabbouleh salad on top of the
    cauliflower rice, top with the roasted salmon
    and the rest of the feta cheese. Drizzle the basil
    dressing over the top and serve.

Avocado, Chicken and Chorizo Salad

Preparation Time: 20 Minutes/Servings: 2 Servings

Nutritional Value: Fat: 24 grams/Fiber: 6 grams/Protein: 42 grams/Calories: 475

Ingredients

- 2 chicken breasts
- 1 teaspoon of coconut oil
- 2 ounces of chorizo sausage
- 1 diced red onion
- 1 cup of sugar snap peas
- ½ an avocado
- 3 tablespoons of pine nuts
- 2 tablespoons of olive oil, separated
- ½ a tablespoon of red wine vinegar
- 1 tablespoon of soy sauce
- 5 ounces of parsley with stalks removed
- 5 ounces of coriander with stalks removed
- 2 tablespoons of mint leaves
- 2 tablespoons of chopped chives
- Salt and pepper

Directions

1. Season the chicken breasts with 1 teaspoon of oil and salt and pepper.

2. Coat a frying pan with the coconut oil and heat over a medium temperature.
3. Fry the chicken breasts until they are cooked all the way through.
4. Lay kitchen paper on a plate and lay the chicken on it to cool down.
5. Once the chicken has cooled down, chop it into bite sized pieces.
6. Chop the chorizo sausage into bite sized pieces and fry on a medium temperature for two minutes.
7. Add one tablespoon of olive oil to a saucepan and cook the onion on low to medium heat for about 5 minutes.
8. Add the red wine vinegar, add the chorizo and stir.
9. Boil some water in a large saucepan.
10. Blanch the sugar snaps for 1 minute and then immediately put them into cold water.
11. Remove them from the water and slice the sugar snap peas in half.
12. Chop the herbs and toss them together in a bowl.
13. Add the sugar snap peas, the chorizo and onion mixture and arrange the avocado, chicken and pine nuts on top.
14. Sprinkle with salt and pepper and serve.

Salmon Wrapped with Prosciutto

Preparation Time: 15 Minutes/Servings: 1 Serving

Nutritional Value: Fat: 21 grams/Fiber: 6 grams/Protein: 38 grams/Calories: 410

Ingredients

- 3 ounces of salmon filet
- 2 thin slices of prosciutto
- ½ a teaspoon of olive oil
- Salt and pepper

Directions

1. Prepare the oven by preheating it to 425 degrees F.
2. Season the salmon with salt and pepper and wrap it in the prosciutto leaving the ends open.
3. Oil a baking pan, lay the wrapped salmon fillets on it and bake for 10 minutes.
4. Once cooked, remove from the oven and serve.

Zucchini Pasta Salad

Preparation Time: Minutes/Servings: 4 Serving

Nutritional Value: Fat: 3.8 grams/Fiber: 3.1 grams/Protein: 1.8 grams/Calories: 76

Ingredients

- 3 spiralled zucchinis
- 3 tablespoons of cooking oil
- ½ a tablespoon of lemon juice
- ¼ teaspoon of garlic powder
- ¼ teaspoon of sea salt
- ⅛ teaspoon of black pepper
- 6 slices of crumbled bacon
- 1 ½ cups of grape tomatoes sliced in half
- 1 teaspoon of rosemary

Directions

1. Whisk the oil, lemon, juice and seasoning in a bowl.
2. Use a spiralizer to turn the zucchini into spaghetti.
3. Combine the zucchini, tomatoes, bacon, rosemary and some oil, toss to combine and serve.

Green Bean Casserole

Preparation Time: 45 Minutes/Serves: 9 Servings

Nutritional Value: Fat: 1.9 grams/Fiber: 3.3 grams/Protein: 4.1 grams/Calories: 191

Ingredients

- 10 Ritz crackers, unsalted
- 3 tablespoons of unsalted butter
- 2 tablespoons of all-purpose flour
- 1 teaspoon of sugar
- 1 cup of sour cream
- ¾ cup of sharp cheddar cheese finely shredded
- 6 cups of frozen green beans, French style
- Cooking spray

Preparation

1. Prepare the oven by heating it to 350 degrees F.
2. Spray a casserole dish with cooking spray.
3. In a small bowl, crush the crackers and set it to one side.
4. Over medium temperature melt 2 tablespoons of butter in a medium frying pan.

5. Add the flour and stir for one minute.

6. Add the cheddar cheese, sour cream and sugar and stir to combine.

7. Add the green beans and stir to combine.

8. Pour the mixture into the casserole dish.

9. Melt 1 tablespoon of butter in the microwave.

10. Pour the butter over the crushed crackers and then sprinkle them on top of the casserole.

11. Bake until the top becomes golden brown, this should take 30 minutes.

Roasted Cauliflower and Carrot Salad

Preparation Time: 35 Minutes/Serves: 8 Servings

Nutritional Value: Fat: 6.1 grams/Fiber: 2.6 grams/Protein: 1.7 grams/Calories: 82.1

Ingredients

- ½ a cup of pomegranate seeds
- 6 cups of baby leaf lettuce
- ¼ teaspoon of black pepper
- ¼ teaspoon of salt (optional)
- ¼ teaspoon of yellow mustard
- 1 ½ tablespoons of maple syrup
- 3 tablespoons of unseasoned rice vinegar
- 1 tablespoon of Italian seasoning blend
- 6 tablespoons of olive oil
- 1 medium diced onion
- 1 large turnip, skin removed and sliced into bite sized chunks
- 5 medium carrots, peeled and cut into bite sized chunks
- 1 small head of cauliflower

Directions

1. Prepare the oven by heating it to 425 degrees F.
2. In a large bowl, combine the onions, turnips, carrots, cauliflower, three tablespoons of olive oil, Italian seasoning blend. Toss to combine.
3. Spread the vegetables out onto the baking tray and put them in the onion for 20 minutes.
4. While the vegetables are cooking, start making the dressing by adding the rest of the olive oil, mustard, maple syrup, rice vinegar and salt and pepper into a bowl. Whisk together thoroughly.
5. Remove the tray from the oven, toss the vegetables and bake for a further 15 minutes, make sure the vegetables are tender before removing them from the oven.
6. Arrange the salad in a bowl and toss with the dressing.
7. Arrange the salad onto plates, top with the roasted vegetables, sprinkle the pomegranate seeds over the top and serve straight away.

Potato, Green Beans and Sheet Pan Chicken Dinner

Preparation Time: 45 Minutes/Serves: 4 Servings

Nutritional Value: Fat: 15.4 grams/Fiber: 2.6 grams/Protein: 39.1 grams/Calories: 374.1

Ingredients

- 1 tablespoon of Italian dressing dry mix
- 4 tablespoons of unsalted butter
- 10 ounces of frozen green beans
- 16 ounces of chicken, sliced into thin strips
- 3 cups of red potatoes, peeled and chopped
- Cooking spray

Directions

1. Prepare the oven by heating it to 400 degrees F.
2. Boil the potatoes for 10 minutes in a large pan of water.
3. Drain the water from the potatoes, refill the pan and boil again until the potatoes become tender, this should take around 10 minutes.
4. Drain the water from the potatoes and set them to one side.
5. Spray a baking tray with cooking spray and arrange the chicken on one end of the tray.
6. Arrange the green beans next to the chicken.

7. Arrange the potatoes next to the green beans.

8. Melt the butter in the microwave and pour it over the food on the tray.

9. Sprinkle the Italian dressing dry mix over the top and roast for 30 minutes.

10. Once cooked, remove from the oven, divide onto plates and serve.

Vegetables with Roasted Rosemary Chicken

Preparation Time: 45 Minutes/Serves: 4 Servings

Nutritional Value: Fat: 4.7 grams/Fiber: 2.7 grams/Protein: 6.1 grams/Calories: 138.7

Ingredients

- 1 tablespoon of dried rosemary
- 4 chicken breasts with the skin and bone
- ½ a teaspoon of ground black pepper
- 1 tablespoon of olive oil
- 8 cloves of crushed garlic
- 1 large red onion, chopped
- ½ a medium bell pepper, chopped
- 1 chopped medium carrot
- 2 medium zucchinis sliced into ½ inch thick rounds

Directions

1. Prepare the oven by heating it to 375 degrees F.
2. In a roasting pan, combine the vegetables, garlic and season with the black pepper.
3. Roast the vegetables for 10 minutes.
4. Pull the skin up on the chicken rub the rosemary and black pepper onto the flesh. Put

the skin back and season the chicken with more rosemary and black pepper.

5. Take the baking pan out of the oven and arrange the chicken on top of the vegetables and bake for around 35 minutes.

6. Once cooked, remove from the oven and serve.

Garden Vegetables and Pork Chops

Preparation Time: 35 Minutes/Serves: 4 Servings

Nutritional Value: Fat: 22.6 grams/Fiber: 5.7 grams/Protein: 30.3 grams/Calories: 520.4

Ingredients

- 4 pork chops
- ½ a cup of yellow onion
- 1 chopped red medium bell pepper
- 1 chopped medium carrot
- 1 chopped yellow medium squash
- 1 cup of chopped eggplant
- 4 sprigs of fresh thyme
- 1 bay leaf
- ½ a teaspoon of pepper
- ½ a teaspoon of salt
- 2 tablespoons of minced garlic
- 2 tablespoons of chopped fresh basil
- 3 tablespoons of olive oil

Directions

1. In a small bowl, combine the thyme, bay leaf, salt, pepper, garlic, basil and olive oil and whisk to combine.
2. Place the eggplant, squash, carrot, bell pepper and onions in a large bowl.

3. Drizzle half of the contents in the small bowl over the vegetables and toss to combine.

4. Arrange the pork chops in the bowl and toss with the rest of the olive oil mixture. Stir to combine, put a lid over the bowl and leave it in the fridge overnight.

5. The next day, prepare the oven by heating it to 400 degrees F.

6. Remove the bowl from the fridge and place the contents onto a baking tray.

7. Bake for 20 minutes, make sure the pork is tender before you remove it from the oven.

Cream of Zucchini

Preparation Time: 25 Minutes/Servings: 5 Serving

Nutritional Value: Fat: 4.9 grams/Fiber: 2.4 grams/Protein: 1.6 grams/Calories: 78.7

Ingredients

- 1 medium chopped onion
- 1 tablespoon of butter
- ½ a teaspoon of sea salt
- 4 medium zucchini, chopped
- 4 cups of vegetable broth
- ½ a cup of heavy cream
- Freshly ground nutmeg

Directions

1. Melt the butter in a medium sized saucepan over medium heat.
2. Add the onion and salt and stir until the onion becomes translucent.
3. Add the zucchini and the broth to the onion mix, turn up the heat and let it boil, and then turn it down the temperature to low and leave it to simmer for 15 minutes until the zucchini becomes tender.

4. Pour the soup into a food processor and blend until it becomes smooth.

5. Pour the soup back into the saucepan, add the cream and then heat on a low temperature.

6. Add some salt, pepper and nutmeg, stir to combine, scoop into bowls and serve.

Stuffed Bell Peppers

Preparation Time: 1 hour/Servings: Serving

Nutritional Value: Fat: 10 grams/Fiber: 5 grams/Protein: 25 grams/Calories: 90

Ingredients

- 1 pound of ground beef
- 4 large bell peppers
- 1 tablespoon of olive oil
- ¼ cup of barbeque sauce
- 2 cups of cauliflower rice
- 1 teaspoon of salt, divided
- ½ a teaspoon of black pepper, divided
- 1 teaspoon of oregano
- 2 cloves of garlic, pressed for juice
- Grated cheddar cheese
- ¼ cup of chopped onion
- Salt and pepper

Directions

1. Prepare the oven by heating it to 400 degrees F.
2. Wash the peppers, slice off the tops and keep them because you will put them back on later.

Remove the seeds and throw them away, season with salt and pepper.

3. Heat the oil in a saucepan and sauté the onions and garlic until they become fragrant.

4. Add the beef and half of the salt and pepper as well as the oregano.

5. Cook the beef until it starts to brown.

6. Add the barbeque sauce, the cauliflower rice and the rest of the salt and pepper. Stir to combine and cook for a further 2 minutes.

7. Stuff the peppers with the mixture, put the tops back on, wrap them in foil and bake for 1 hour.

8. Take the peppers out of the oven, unwrap the foil, remove the tops and add the cheese. Put the peppers back in the oven (minus the foil) for 10 minutes.

9. Remove from the oven and serve.

Pesto Salmon

Preparation Time: 25 Minutes/Servings: 4 Servings

Nutritional Value: Fat: 17.2 grams/Fiber: 5.9 grams/Protein: 50.1 grams/Calories: 400.4

Ingredients

- Four 3-ounce salmon fillets
- 1 cup of fresh cilantro
- 3 tablespoons of lime juice
- Salt and pepper
- 3 cloves of garlic
- 2 tablespoons of olive oil

Directions

1. Prepare the oven by preheating it to 475 degrees F.
2. Line a baking tray with parchment paper.
1. For the pesto, blend the garlic, olive oil, cilantro and lime juice in a food processor.
2. Season the salmon fillets with salt and pepper.
3. Heat the olive oil in a frying pan and cook the salmon for 5 minutes.
4. Arrange the salmon on the baking tray and bake for 12 minutes.
5. Once cooked, remove the salmon from the oven, pour the pesto over the top and serve.

Cuban Roast Pork

Preparation Time: 18 hours/Servings: 4 Serving

Nutritional Value: Fat: 9.4 grams/Fiber: 0.9 grams/Protein: 42.5 grams/Calories: 280.1

Ingredients

- 4 boneless pork shoulders
- 2 teaspoons of ground cumin
- 4 teaspoons of fine salt
- 1 teaspoon of pepper
- ¼ cup of olive oil
- 5 sprigs of fresh oregano
- 1 large red onion, diced
- 4 cloves of minced garlic
- The juice of 1 orange
- The juice of 2 lemons
- Cooked brown rice

Directions

1. Arrange the pork shoulders in a large bowl and season them with salt and pepper.
2. Combine the rest of the ingredients in a food processor and blend until combined.
3. Pour the blended ingredients over the meat, cover and put it in the fridge overnight.

4. The next day, arrange the pork shoulders in a pressure cooker or a crockpot, pour the marinade over the top. If cooking in a pressure cooker, cook on high for 40 minutes, if cooking in a crockpot, cook on low for 8 hours.
5. Whilst the pork shoulders are cooking, preheat the oven to 425 degrees F.
6. Once the pork shoulders are cooked, arrange them onto a baking tray and roast for 30 minutes until they become golden and crispy.
7. Continue cooking the juice for 20 minutes.
8. Remove the pork shoulders from the oven, shred it and pour the marinade over the top.
9. Serve with brown rice.

Pimiento Cheese Meatballs with Zucchini Pasta

Preparation Time: 35 Minutes/Servings: 12 meatballs

Nutritional Value: Fat: 52 grams/Fiber: 1 gram/Protein: 41 grams/Calories: 651

Ingredients

- Spiralised zucchini noodles
- 2 ounces of cream cheese
- 2 cups of Monterey cheese
- 2 cups of sharp cheddar cheese
- 1 teaspoon of grated onion
- ⅛ teaspoon of garlic powder
- 3 tablespoons of mayonnaise
- 3 tablespoons of pimientos, chopped, drained
- Salt and pepper
- 1 ½ cups of finely chopped roasted pecans

Directions

1. Blend the cream in a food processor until it becomes smooth.
2. Add the Monterey cheese, cheddar cheese, mayonnaise, pimientos, onion, garlic powder, salt and pepper and pulse.
3. Scrape into a bowl, cover and refrigerate for 30 minutes.

4. Place the pecans in a medium bowl, roll the cheese mixture into 1-inch balls and coat them with pecans.

5. Boil or microwave the zucchini noodles until soft, spoon onto plates and serve with the meatballs.

Tuna Casserole

Preparation Time: 35 Minutes/Servings: 3 Serving

Nutritional Value: Fat: 7 grams/Fiber: 5 grams/Protein: 16 grams/Calories: 450

Ingredients

- 2 small cans of tuna, drained
- ⅓ cup of mayo
- 1 tablespoon of Dijon mustard
- ¼ cup of chopped onion
- ¼ teaspoon of salt
- ¼ teaspoon of pepper
- ¼ teaspoon of cayenne pepper
- ½ a cup of shredded gruyere cheese, divided
- ¼ cup of chopped parsley

Directions

1. Prepare the oven by preheating it to 400 degrees F.
2. In a medium sized bowl, combine the tuna, mayonnaise, mustard, ¼ cup of gruyere cheese, salt, pepper and cayenne pepper.
3. Place in a casserole dish and scatter the rest of the cheese over the top.
4. Bake for 15 minutes.
5. Remove from the oven, arrange onto plates, sprinkle with parsley and serve.

Bacon Cheeseburger Bake

Preparation Time: 25 Minutes/Servings: 4 Servings

Nutritional Value: Fat: 27.9 grams/Fiber: 0 grams/Protein: 30.4 grams/Calories: 391

Ingredients

- 1 pound of hamburger
- 1 cup of chopped onion
- 2 cloves of minced garlic
- 1 teaspoon of Worcestershire sauce
- 2 ounces of cream cheese
- 1 teaspoon of olive oil
- 2 eggs
- 1-2 tablespoons of mustard
- ½ a cup of heavy whipping cream
- 1 cup of shredded cheddar cheese, divided
- 1 cup of shredded white cheddar cheese
- Salt and pepper
- 1 teaspoon of all-purpose seasoning
- 3 slices of crumbled bacon
- 1 kosher pickle sliced into pieces

Directions

1. Prepare the oven by preheating it to 350 degrees F.
2. In a frying pan heat the oil and cook the hamburger meat, garlic, onions, salt, pepper and the all-purpose seasoning and stir to combine.
3. Add the Worcestershire sauce, and the cream cheese and cook until the cheese has melted.
4. Take the frying pan off the heat.
5. In a medium bowl combine the eggs, cheeses, heavy cream and mustard and whisk together thoroughly.
6. Grease a baking dish and transfer the hamburger mixture into it.
7. Add the bacon and pickles and stir to combine.
8. Smear the heavy cream mixture over the top.
9. Sprinkle the remaining cheese over the top.
10. Bake for 15-20 minutes or until the cheese starts to bubble.
11. Remove from the oven and serve.

Lamb Sliders

Preparation Time: 35 Minutes/Servings: 8 sliders

Nutritional Value: Fat: 31 grams/Fiber: 5 grams/Protein: 36 grams/Calories: 540

Ingredients

- 1 pound of ground lamb
- 1 zested lemon
- ½ a teaspoon of ground black pepper
- ¼ yellow onion
- 2 cloves of minced garlic
- 2 teaspoons of fresh oregano leaves
- ½ a teaspoon of sea salt
- Whole-wheat burger buns
- 8 slices of tomatoes
- 8 lettuce leaves
- Ketchup
- Mustard

Directions

1. Put the lamb in a bowl and season it with salt and pepper.
2. Add the diced onions, minced garlic, oregano leaves, and lemon zest. Mix until the meat is evenly coated.

3. Preheat the grill to medium-high heat.

4. Form 8 patties out of the mixture.

5. Grill the burgers for 4 minutes on each side.

6. Once cooked arrange the burgers onto buns, top with lettuce, tomatoes, ketchup and mayonnaise.

Bacon Wrapped Meatloaf

Preparation Time: Minutes/Servings: 4 Servings

Nutritional Value: Fat: 31.5 grams/Fiber: 0.7 grams/Protein: 21.1 grams/Calories: 417.5

Ingredients

- 1 tablespoon of extra virgin olive oil
- 1 chopped medium onion
- 1 chopped celery stalk
- 3 cloves of minced garlic
- 2 eggs
- 1 teaspoon of dried oregano
- 1 teaspoon of chili powder
- ½ a cup of almond flour
- 2 pounds of ground beef
- Salt and pepper
- 1 cup of shredded cheddar cheese
- ¼ cup of grated parmesan cheese
- 1 tablespoon of low sodium soy sauce
- 6 strips of bacon

Directions

1. Prepare the oven by preheating it to 400 degrees F.
2. Grease a medium sized baking dish.

3. Heat the oil in a frying pan and sauté the onion, celery, garlic, oregano and chili powder. Cook until fragrant and then allow the mixture to cook down.

4. Combine the remainder of the ingredients in a large bowl, transfer the contents of the frying pan into the bowl, stir to combine and then shape into a meatloaf.

5. Wrap the bacon around the meatloaf and bake in the oven for approximately 1 hour.

6. Remove from the oven and serve with a side dish of your choice.

Salmon with Lemon

Preparation Time: 35 Minutes/Servings: Serving

Nutritional Value: Fat: 19.8 grams/Fiber: 1.6 grams/Protein: 20.3 grams/Calories: 283.2

Ingredients

- Two 3-ounce salmon filets
- 1 tablespoon of olive oil
- Salt and pepper
- Half a stick of butter
- 1 zested lemon
- A handful of asparagus

Directions

1. Prepare the oven by preheating it to 400 degrees F.
2. Grease a baking tray with olive oil.
3. Lay the salmon skin side down and sprinkle with salt and pepper.
4. Thinly slice the lemon and arrange it on the salmon.
5. Thinly slice the butter and arrange it on the lemon.
6. Bake for 30 minutes.
7. Once cooked, removed from the oven and serve with asparagus.

Tropical Frozen Chocolate Monkey

Preparation time: 15 Minutes /Serves: 2 servings

Nutritional Value: Fat: 16.7 grams/Fiber: 2.7 grams/Protein: 15.5 grams/Calories: 533

Ingredients

- 2 frozen bananas
- 2 tablespoons of coconut oil
- 2 tablespoons of cacao powder
- 1 tablespoon of cacao nibs
- 2 tablespoons of chia seeds
- 2 cups of coconut milk

Directions

1. Blend all the ingredients until smooth except the chia seeds in a food processor.
2. Add the chia seeds and pulse a few times.
3. Transfer into bowls and serve.

Summer Fruit Mixed Salad

Preparation time: 15 Minutes /Serves: 4 servings

Nutritional Value: Fat: 0.2 grams/Fiber: 3.4 grams/Protein: 1 gram/Calories: 84

Ingredients

- 1 chopped pitted peach
- 1 chopped pitted nectarine
- ½ a cup of cherries, seeds and stems removed
- ½ a cup of blueberries
- The juice and zest of one lemon
- 1 teaspoon of chopped mint
- 1 heaping tablespoon of coconut butter

Directions

1. Combine all the ingredients in a large bowl and toss to combine.
2. Divide into bowls and serve.

Alkaline Macaroons

Preparation time: 5 Hours /Serves: 20 macaroons

Nutritional Value: Fat: 3 grams/Fiber: 0 grams/Protein: 2 grams/Calories: 90

Ingredients

- 1 cup of raw almonds
- 1 cup of coconut flakes, unsweetened
- 1 cup of apricots
- 3 teaspoons of cardamom
- ½ a teaspoon of vanilla extract

Directions

1. Transfer all ingredients into a food processor and blend for 2 minutes until smooth.
2. Use your hands to mold the batter into macaroons.
3. Arrange the macaroons onto dehydrator sheets
4. Set the dehydrator to 115 degrees F and dehydrate for 3-4 hours.
5. Serve with coconut butter or almond butter.
6. If you don't have a dehydrator you can heat them in a toaster oven, or you can eat them raw.

Ice-cream flavoured with vanilla cardamom

Preparation time: 40 minutes/Serves: 4 people

Nutritional Value: Fat: 4.5 grams/Fiber: 0 grams/Protein: 1 grams/Calories: 80

Ingredients

- 2 cups of coconut milk
- 2 tablespoons of vegetable glycerine
- ¾ teaspoons of powdered stevia
- ¾ teaspoons of ground cardamom ideally from 5 to 6 fresh green pods
- 1 teaspoon of vanilla extract (alcohol free)
- 1/8 teaspoon of salt

Directions

1. Crush the cardamom pods open with the bottom of a saucepan. Take the seeds out of the pod shells and reserve the shells. Using a mortar and pestle, coffee grinder or a spice grinder, grind the seeds. Put the pod shells and the ground seeds to one side.

2. Cut the vanilla bean in half lengthwise. Using a knife, scoop the seeds out and set the pod and the seeds to one side.

3. Pour the coconut milk, powdered stevia, vegetable glycerine, seeds, pod, ground

cardamom, salt, vanilla seeds and pod into a saucepan. Mix together thoroughly and allow to simmer. Take the pan off the cooker and steep for 30 minutes. Sieve the mixture into a bowl and press on the pulp to extract the liquid. Set the bowl into the refrigerator and allow it to chill for 3 to 4 hours.

4. Transfer the cream mixture into an ice-cream maker and prepare as per the manufacturer's directions. It should take approximately 20 minutes for the ice-cream to set. Spoon the ice-cream into a freezer friendly container and freeze for 3 to four hours.

Sugar Free Eggnog

Preparation time: 10 minutes/Serves: 4 people

Nutritional Value: Fat: 9.76 grams/Fiber: 0.53 grams/Protein: 4.63 grams/Calories: 123

Ingredients

- 1 can of coconut milk at room temperature (12 ounces)
- ¼ cup of almond milk (unsweetened)
- 2 large eggs
- 1 to 2 packets of stevia
- ½ teaspoon of fresh grated nutmeg
- ¼ teaspoon of cinnamon

Directions

1. Pour the almond milk, coconut milk, vanilla, eggs, nutmeg, stevia and cinnamon into a blender. Process the mixture on a high speed until it becomes frothy.
2. Chill by adding ice or setting it in the fridge.
3. Transfer into glasses and sprinkle cinnamon over the top.

Vanilla coconut custard

Preparation time: 40 minutes/Serves: 4 people

Nutritional Value: Fat: 54 grams/Fiber: 2.8 grams/Protein: 12 grams/Calories: 690

Ingredients

- 4 large egg yolks
- 1 ½ cups of coconut milk divided
- One piece of vanilla bean (2 inches)
- 1 teaspoon of powdered stevia
- Flaked coconut

Directions

1. Preheat the oven to 350 degrees F.
2. Cut the vanilla bean in half lengthwise and scrape out the seeds with a knife.
3. Separate the egg yolks into a medium bowl and whisk together thoroughly. In another medium sized bowl add ¾ cups of coconut milk, put a strainer over the bowl and set it to one side.
4. Heat a saucepan over medium heat, add the stevia, ¾ cups of coconut milk, vanilla seeds and bean. Heat the mixture until it starts steaming, do not allow it to simmer.

Pour the mixture into the bowl of egg yolks and whisk together thoroughly.

5. Sieve the mixture into the bowl of coconut milk and whisk together thoroughly.

6. Pour the mixture into 4 custard cups; put the cups into a deep pan. Fill the pan halfway up the custard cups with hot water that hasn't been boiled. Place foil over the pan and seal tightly. Bake for 25 to 30 minutes until the edges are firm but the center is soft.

7. Take the custard cups out of the pan and allow them to cool. Sprinkle the flaked coconut over the top, serve chilled or at room temperature.

No-Bake Peanut Butter Cookies

Preparation Time: 40 Minutes/Servings: 12 cookies

Nutritional Value: Fat: 6.5 grams/Fiber: 1.1 grams/Protein: 2.6 grams/Calories: 133

Ingredients

- 1 ⅓ cups of creamy peanut butter
- 1 teaspoon of erythritol
- 2 teaspoons of vanilla extract
- 2 tablespoons of unsweetened cocoa powder
- 2 cups of unsweetened coconut flakes
- 2 tablespoons of melted butter

Directions

1. Line a baking sheet with parchment paper.
2. Combine the peanut butter, vanilla, melted butter, coconut flakes, and cocoa powder and stir well.
3. Scoop the batter onto the baking tray into 12 cookie shapes.
4. Freeze for 30 minutes and serve.

Chocolate Mug Cake

Preparation Time: 7 Minutes/Servings: Serving

Nutritional Value: Fat: 47 grams/Fiber: 8 grams/Protein: 23 grams/Calories: 1117

Ingredients

- 2 tablespoons of butter
- 1 tablespoon of coconut oil
- 2 teaspoons of unsweetened cocoa powder
- 3 tablespoons of almond flour
- 3 tablespoons of erythritol
- 1 egg

Directions

1. Add the butter and the coconut oil to a mug, heat until melted and stir.
2. Add all the dry ingredients and whisk together thoroughly.
3. Cook in the microwave for 2 minutes.

Coconut Macadamia Bars

Preparation Time: 1 hour 10 Minutes/Servings: Serving16

Nutritional Value: Fat: 19.3 grams/Fiber: 2.1 grams/Protein: 3.1 grams/Calories: 199

Ingredients for The Crust

- 1 ¼ cups of flour
- ⅓ cups of sugar free liquid sweetener
- ¼ teaspoon of salt
- ¼ cup of butter

Ingredients for The Filing

- ¼ cup of butter
- ½ a cup of sugar-free liquid sweetener
- ½ a cup of coconut cream
- 1 ⅓ cups of coconut flakes
- ¾ cups of macadamia nuts, chopped
- 1 egg yolk
- ½ a teaspoon of vanilla extract

Directions for The Crust

1. Prepare the oven by preheating it to 350 degrees F.
2. In a food processor, combine the flour, sweetener and salt and blend.

3. Add the butter and pulse into fine chunks.

4. Press the mixture into a baking pan and leave it to sit for 15 minutes.

Directions for The Filling

1. Melt the butter in a small saucepan and add the coconut cream, sugar and liquid sweetener, whisk to combine.

2. Add the coconut flakes, macadamia nuts, egg yolk, and vanilla extract and whisk to combine.

3. Pour the mixture on top of the crust and bake for 40 minutes.

4. Once cooked, remove the baking dish from the oven and leave it to cool down before slicing into bars.

Lemon Bars

Preparation Time: 55 Minutes/Servings: 36 Servings

Nutritional Value: Fat: 5.8 grams/Fiber: 0.5 grams/Protein: 1.6 grams/Calories: 126

Ingredients

- ½ a cup of melted butter
- 1 2/4 cups of almond flour divided into half
- 1 cup of powdered erythritol, divided into half
- 3 medium lemons
- 3 eggs

Directions

1. Prepare the oven by heating it to 350 degrees F.
2. Mix the butter, 1 cup of almond flour, ¼ cups of erythritol and a pinch of salt in a small bowl.
3. Line a baking pan with parchment paper and press the mixture into it.
4. In a medium sized bowl, combine the eggs, ¾ erythritol, ¾ cup of almond flour and salt.
5. Pour the filling onto the crust and bake for 25 minutes.

6. Once cooked, remove the baking pan from the
    oven and freeze for 20 minutes before slicing
    and serving.

Caramel Salted Cake Bombs

Preparation Time: 1 hour 10 Minutes/Servings: 12 Servings

Nutritional Value: Fat: 2 grams/Fiber: 0.4 grams/Protein: 2.2 grams/Calories: 40

Ingredients for The Cake

- 2.75 cups of almond flour
- 1.25 cups of confectioners' sugar
- 0.5 cups of unsweetened cocoa powder
- 2 teaspoons of gluten-free baking powder
- ½ a teaspoon of salt
- 6 large eggs
- ½ a cup of melted butter
- 1 cup of pumpkin puree
- 1 tablespoon of vanilla extract

Ingredients for The Caramel

- ½ a cup of heavy cream
- ½ a cup of unsalted butter
- ½ a cup of Swerve brown sugar substitute
- 1 teaspoon of vanilla extract

Ingredients for The Glaze

- 9 ounces of sugar free chocolate chip cookies
- 1 tablespoon of coconut oil
- Sea salt

Directions

1. Prepare the oven by preheating it to 325 degrees F.
2. Line a cake pan with parchment paper.
3. Combine all the cake ingredients in a bowl and whisk until smooth.
4. Transfer the batter to the cake pan and bake for 55 minutes.
5. Make the caramel by combining all the ingredients in a saucepan, stir to combine and cook over medium temperature for 5-6 minutes.
6. Once the cake is cooked, remove it from the oven and crumble it into small pieces.
7. Pour the caramel over the crumbled cake.
8. Line a baking sheet with parchment paper.
9. Roll the caramel cake into small balls and arrange them on the parchment paper.
10. Put the baking sheet into the oven and freeze.
11. Combine the chips and the coconut oil in a bowl and microwave until soft.
12. Dip the balls into the mixture.
13. Sprinkle the sea salt over the top and freeze for 10 minutes before serving.

Raspberry Dream Cheesecake

Preparation Time: 50 Minutes/Servings: 6 Slices

Nutritional Value: Fat: 72 grams/Fiber: 2 grams/Protein: 11 grams/Calories: 648

Ingredients for The Crust

- 2 cups of almond flour
- ⅓ cup of melted butter
- 3 tablespoons of powdered sweetener
- 1 teaspoon of vanilla

Ingredients for The Filling

- Four 3-ounce packages of softened cream cheese
- 1.5 cups of powdered sweetener
- 4 eggs
- 1 tablespoon of lemon juice
- ¼ tablespoon of lemon zest
- 1 teaspoon of vanilla extract
- 1 cup of fresh raspberries
- Raspberries for garnish
- 2 tablespoons of powdered sweetener

Directions

1. Prepare the oven by preheating it to 350 degrees F.

2. Grease a baking pan with butter and line it with parchment paper.
3. Combine the almond flour, butter, sweetener and vanilla extract in a food processor until the ingredients form into large sticky crumbs.
4. Make the crust by sticking the crumbs down into the baking pan and bake for 10 minutes.
5. Turn the oven down to 325 degrees F.
6. Combine the sweetener and the cream cheese in a bowl and whisk until smooth.
7. Add the eggs one at a time until a batter like consistency has been achieved.
8. Add the lemon juice, lemon zest, and teaspoon of vanilla.
9. Add the batter to the crust and wrap the pan in foil.
10. Combine the raspberries and 2 tablespoons of sweetener in a food processor and blend until the ingredients turn into a puree.
11. Set aside some of the puree for garnish and fold the remainder into the pan.
12. Bake for 75 minutes.
13. Once cooked, remove the cheesecake from the oven and leave it to cool down.
14. Garnish with the puree and some fresh raspberries and serve.

Swiss Roll Cake

Preparation Time: Minutes/Servings: 12 Servings

Nutritional Value: Fat: 36 grams/Fiber: 15 grams/Protein: 8 grams/Calories: 391 grams

Ingredients for the Cake

- 1 cup of almond flour
- ¼ cup of psyllium husk powder
- ¼ cup of cocoa powder
- 1 teaspoon of baking powder
- 3 eggs
- ¼ cup of coconut milk
- 4 tablespoons of melted butter
- ¼ cup of sour cream
- ¼ cup of erythritol
- 1 teaspoon of vanilla

Ingredients for The Frosting

- 8 ounces of cream cheese
- ¼ cup of sour cream
- 8 tablespoons of butter
- 1 teaspoon of vanilla extract
- ¼ cup of erythritol
- ¼ cup of liquid Stevia

Directions

1. Prepare the oven by preheating it to 350 degrees.
2. Grease a baking pan and put it to one side.
3. To make the cake, in a mixing bowl, combine the almond flour, psyllium husk powder, baking powder, and erythritol, whisk together thoroughly.
4. In a microwave safe bowl, melt 4 tablespoons of butter in the microwave.
5. Remove the butter from the microwave and add 3 eggs, ¼ cup of sour cream and whisk to combine.
6. Add 4 tablespoons of coconut milk and continue to whisk.
7. Pour the batter into the greased baking pan and bake for 13 minutes.
8. Once the cake has set, remove it from the oven and set it to one side to cool down.
9. To make the filling, combine 8 tablespoons of butter, 8 ounces of cream cheese, ¼ cup of erythritol. ¼ cup of sour cream, 1 teaspoon of vanilla extract, and ¼ teaspoon of liquid Stevia to a bowl and combine the ingredients until they turn into a smooth cream.
10. Spoon the cream onto the cake and roll the cake to form a swiss roll.
11. Cut into slices and serve.

Peanut Butter Cookies

Preparation Time: 30 Minutes/Servings: 18 cookies

Nutritional Value: Fat: 8.5 grams/Fiber: 1.6 grams/Protein: 2.4 grams/Calories: 97 grams

Ingredients

- ⅓ cup of flour
- ¼ cup of flaxseed meal
- 1 tablespoon of heavy whipping cream
- ½ a cup of natural peanut butter
- ⅓ cup of erythritol
- 1 tablespoon of baking powder
- ¼ teaspoon of baking soda
- 5 tablespoons of salted butter
- 1 egg

Directions

1. Prepare the oven by preheating it to 350 degrees F.
2. Cover a large cookie sheet with parchment paper.
3. In a large mixing bowl, combine the heavy cream, butter and peanut butter and whisk to combine.

4. Add the baking powder, baking soda, coconut flour, erythritol and flax seed meal into the mixture and whisk to combine.
5. Add the egg and whisk to combine.
6. Use your hands to form 18 rounded cookies and arrange them onto the cookie sheet.
7. Bake for 15 minutes, once cooked, remove from the oven and serve.

Coffee Time Cookies

Preparation Time: Minutes/Servings: 10 Cookies

Nutritional Value: Fat: 17.1 grams/Fiber: 1.4 grams/Protein: 3.9 grams/Calories: 167

Ingredients

- 1 ½ cups of almond flour
- ½ a teaspoon of baking soda
- ½ a teaspoon of salt
- ½ a cup of unsalted butter
- 1 tablespoon of instant coffee grounds
- 1 teaspoon of instant coffee grounds
- 2 eggs
- ⅓ cup of erythritol
- 17 drops of liquid Stevia
- 1 ½ teaspoons of vanilla extract
- ¼ teaspoon of cinnamon

Directions

1. Prepare your oven by preheating it to 350 degrees F.
2. Cover a large cookie tray with parchment paper.

3. In a large mixing bowl, combine the almond flour, baking soda, salt, ground coffee and cinnamon and stir together thoroughly.

4. Separate the egg whites and the yolks.

5. Add the butter to another bowl and use an electric hand mixer to whip it into a creamy consistency.

6. Add ⅓ cup of erythritol and continue whipping until the butter turns white.

7. Add the egg yolks and continue to whisk until combined.

8. Add half of the dry ingredients to the wet ingredients and continue to whip.

9. Add the liquid Stevia and 1 ½ cups of vanilla extract and whisk to combine.

10. Add the rest of the dry ingredients and whisk to combine.

11. Whip the egg whites until stiff peaks are formed and then fold it into the dough.

12. Use your hands to form 10 cookies out of the dough and set them onto the baking sheet.

13. Bake the cookies for approximately 12 minutes.

14. Once cooked, remove them from the oven and serve.

Holiday Ice-cream

Preparation Time: Minutes/Servings: 1 Serving

Nutritional Value: Fat: 12 grams/Fiber: 0 grams/Protein: 0 grams/Calories: 131

Ingredients

- 1 pint of heavy cream
- 2 tablespoons of dark chocolate chips
- 1.8 ounces of unsweetened shredded coconut
- 1.8 ounces of chopped strawberries
- 2 tablespoons of Stevia

Directions

1. Combine the stevia and cream into a medium sized mixing bowl and whisk together to combine.
2. Fold in the dark chocolate chips, strawberries and coconut.
3. Put the bowl in the freezer and leave it to freeze overnight.
4. When ready to eat, sit the bowl in warm water so that it melts a bit and serve.

Chocolate Chipotle Fat Bombs

Preparation Time: 15 Minutes (1-hour chilling time)/Servings: 12 Fat bombs

Nutritional Value: Fat: 18 grams/Fiber: 0 grams/Protein: 0 grams/Calories: 166

Ingredients

- ¾ cup of coconut oil
- ¼ cup of butter at room temperature
- ¼ cup of cocoa powder
- 2 teaspoons of granulated erythritol
- 1/8 teaspoon of chipotle chili powder

Directions

1. Place a medium saucepan over low heat and combine the coconut oil, butter, cocoa powder, erythritol and chili powder in a pan.
2. Whisk until the ingredients melt and are well mixed, this should take around 3 minutes.
3. Pour the mixture evenly into 12 mini metal or silicone muffin cups.

4. Place the muffin cups into the refrigerator until very firm. This should take around 1 hour.

5. Pop the fat bombs out of the muffin cups and serve.

Cheese Crusted Portobello Mushrooms

Preparation Time: 30 Minutes/Servings: 4 servings

Nutritional Value: Fat: 22 grams/Fiber: 3 grams/Protein: 13 grams/Calories: 282

Ingredients

- ¼ cup of extra virgin olive oil
- 2 tablespoons of balsamic vinegar
- Salt and pepper
- 4 medium portobello mushrooms, stemmed and black gills scooped out
- 1/3 cup of ground almonds
- ¼ cup of shredded Asiago cheese
- 1 tablespoon of freshly chopped basil
- 1 tablespoon of freshly chopped oregano
- 4 ounces of shredded mozzarella cheese

Directions

1. Prepare the oven by preheating it to 400 degrees F.
2. Line a baking sheet with parchment paper and set it to one side.
3. In a medium bowl, stir together the olive oil and balsamic vinegar and season lightly with salt and pepper.

4. Add the mushrooms to the dressing and toss to coat.
5. Place the mushrooms on the baking sheet hollow side up and roast until tender, this should take around 12 minutes.
6. While the mushrooms are roasting, stir together the ground almonds, Asiago cheese, basil, and oregano in a small bowl.
7. Remove the mushrooms from the oven and carefully tip out and discard any liquid collected in the hollows. Evenly divide the mozzarella among the hollows and top with the almond mixture.
8. Bake the mushrooms until the cheese toppings are golden and bubbly, this should take around 5 minutes.
9. Remove the mushrooms from the oven and serve.

Smoked Salmon Deviled Eggs

Preparation Time: 20 Minutes/Servings: 5 Servings

Nutritional Value: Fat: 15 grams/Fiber: 0 grams/Protein: 10 grams/Calories: 179

Ingredients

- 5 large hard-boiled eggs
- ½ a cup of mayonnaise
- 3 ounces of chopped smoked salmon
- ½ a teaspoon of Dijon mustard
- ¼ teaspoon of chopped fresh dill
- Freshly ground black pepper

Directions

1. Half each of the eggs lengthwise and carefully remove the yolks.
2. Place the yolks in a medium bowl.
3. Place the egg whites on a plate hollow side up.
4. Mash the yolks with a fork and stir in the mayonnaise, smoked salmon, mustard and dill until very well mixed.
5. Season the mixture with pepper.
6. Spoon the mixture into the egg white halves and serve.

Jalapeno Lunch Poppers

Preparation Time: 20 Minutes/Servings: 4 Servings

Nutritional Value: Fat: 21 grams/Fiber: 1 gram/Protein: 11 grams/Calories: 245

Ingredients

- 4 large jalapeno peppers
- 4 ounces of cream cheese at room temperature
- 4 ounces of goat cheese at room temperature
- 1 scallion, green parts only, finely chopped
- 2 tablespoons of chopped fresh cilantro
- ¼ teaspoon of garlic powder
- 1/8 teaspoon of red pepper flakes
- ½ a cup of shredded cheddar cheese
- 1 tablespoon of chopped fresh parsley for garnish

Directions

1. Prepare the oven by preheating it to 400 degrees F.
2. Line a baking sheet with parchment paper and set it to one side.
3. Cut the jalapeno peppers in half lengthwise, scoop out the seeds and discard them.

4. Arrange the jalapenos on the prepared baking
    sheet.
5. In a medium bowl, stir together the cream
    cheese, goat cheese, scallion, cilantro, garlic
    powder, and red pepper flakes.
6. Divide the filling evenly between among the
    pepper halves and top each with cheddar
    cheese.
7. Bake until the peppers are softened, the filling
    is bubbly, and the cheese topping is golden
    brown. This should table around 12 to 14
    minutes.
8. Remove from the oven, top with parsley and
    serve.

Pistachio Crusted Goat Cheese

Preparation Time: 20 Minutes/Servings: 4 Servings

Nutritional Value: Fat: 23 grams/Fiber: 2 grams/Protein: 12 grams/Calories: 279

Ingredients

- ¼ cup of almond flour
- 1 large egg beaten with 2 tablespoons of water
- 3 ounces of finely chopped pistachios
- 1 teaspoon of chopped fresh thyme
- 4-ounce log of goat cheese
- 1 tablespoon of extra-virgin olive oil

Directions

1. Place the almond flour on a plate and place the bowl with the beaten egg next to the almond flour. Combine the pistachios and thyme on another plate next to the egg.
2. Cut the goat cheese using a thin thread or wire into 8 equal rounds.
3. Dip a goat cheese round into the almond flour, then the egg, then the pistachios, make sure the goat cheese is completely covered. Do the same with the remaining goat cheese.

4. Heat the olive oil in a large skillet over medium heat and panfry the goat cheese rounds, turning carefully once until lightly browned on both sides.

5. Serve immediately.

CONCLUSION

Intermittent fasting may work amazingly well for some women and not so good for others. The only way to know if it works for you is by giving it a try and listening to your body throughout the process. Easing into intermittent fasting by starting with a shorter fasting window can help with initial symptoms of hunger and discomfort. But if it becomes too uncomfortable, be honest with yourself, accept it and move on.

At the end of the day, nothing can have a greater impact on your health than a diet consisting of real, whole foods, and a lifestyle that prioritizes your physical, emotional and mental well-being.

I hope this book was able to help you discover the right fasting method for you. The next step is to apply what you have learned by creating a fasting plan that works with your current lifestyle and helps you achieve your personal fitness goals.

You should also go for a consultation with your physician in order to get their opinion about your plan to fast. Once you start, make sure you are able to fully commit to it.

I wish you every success on your intermittent fasting journey!